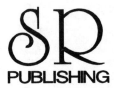

PUBLISHING

Series Editor: Wendy Thompson
Copy Editor: Maura McMillan
Cover design: Veronica Burnett

Notice: The author and the publisher of this volume have taken care
to make certain that all information is correct and compatible with the
standards generally accepted at the time of publication.

Reynolds, Audree

The Skidmore-Roth Outline Series: Medical-Surgical Nursing/Audree
Reynolds

ISBN 1-56930-068-2

1. Nursing-Handbooks, Manuals.
2. Medical-Handbooks, Manuals.

SKIDMORE-ROTH PUBLISHING, INC.
2620 S. Parker Rd., Suite 147
Aurora, CO 80014
303-306-1455

Web address: http://www.skidmore-roth.com

Reviewers

Carol Baxter Zeller, RN, MSN
Instructor
College of Marin
Kentfield, California

Barbara Acello, MS Ed, RN
Innovations in Health Care Consulting
Denton, Texas

Table of Contents

Preface

Using the convenient outline format, readers will be able to focus on the essential rationale underlying the nursing care of adults with common, recurring medical-surgical conditions. With the changes in health care delivery, competent care will be provided in acute care, home health or skilled care setting. The warning signs of evolving serious problems and complications are addressed which will assist the nurse in any setting with the decision of whether to seek referral or transfer to a more acute setting. However, unstable clinical situations which require continuous monitoring and care on a critical care unit are not included in this publication.

This outline was written to provide a concise rationale for nursing care. Units of major physiological dysfunction are subdivided into sections which address anatomical and physiological review, considerations for the elderly client, key point of dysfunction, interventions to improve physiological function and examples of common clinical conditions. The focus is on essential "need to know" content as the basis for safe, competent nursing practice.

Unique features in each unit include focused, head-to-toe assessments which identify typical data observed with common recurring clinical problems. Decision trees provide a schematic of sequence of clinical decision making related to major clinical manifestations. Diagrams of pertinent nursing techniques and equipment clarify often difficult to understand aspects.

It is hoped that this outline will be helpful as we bridge this period of transition in health care delivery. Our goal of professional nursing continues to focus on the provision of competent, caring nursing care regardless of the setting. Our patients and their families will continue to benefit because of our presence and abilities.

Your comments and suggestions are welcome.

Audree Reynolds

unit *1*

NURSING CARE OF ADULTS WITH

Neurological Conditions

This unit addresses common and stable neurological conditions of adults cared for on general medical-surgical nursing units. The management and care of critical and unstable conditions, such as acute increased intracranial pressure, acute head and spinal cord injuries and immediate post-operative craniotomy are not included. Stabilized, intermediate and convalescent management of care is addressed. Clinical situations in which an individual is at risk for developing an acute change in their neurological status are included. Often only subtle clues of neurological dysfunction are noticeable and detected by the providers of daily care. Early detection and prompt initiation of interventions determine the long-term outcome and minimize the development of complications.

SECTION 1: OVERVIEW

The nursing care of adults with neurological dysfunction encompasses a wide variety of pathophysiological conditions. Effective plans for care are based upon an understanding of the normal functioning of the nervous system. Often only subtle clues of neurological dysfunction are noticeable and detected by the nurse at the bedside.

Anatomical Considerations

1. A network of integrated structures are responsible for the body's ability to interact with surroundings and to regulate internal physiological functions. The central nervous system (CNS) includes the brain and spinal cord enclosed in rigid bony compartments, the skull and vertebral column.

2. Three coverings (meninges) protect the brain from external injury: dura mater, arachnoid mater and pia mater. A fold in the meninges (tentorium) at the lower back of the brain separates the cerebrum from the brain stem and cerebellum.

3. Cerebospinal fluid (CSF) circulates around the brain and spinal cord and protects it from injury. It also serves as a fluid cushion and supports the weight of the brain. Approximately 600 ml of CSF is formed each day in the lateral ventricles of the cerebrum. It circulates within the subarachnoid space and is reabsorbed back into the venous system on the surface of the brain.

4. The peripheral nervous system (PNS) includes cranial and spinal nerves. Afferent (sensory) nerve pathways carry impulses toward both nervous systems. Efferent (motor) nerve pathways carry impulses away from the nervous systems.

5. Spinal nerves exit the spinal cord between vertebra. Each nerve has a specific destination in the skeletomuscular system. The areas of nerve innervation on the surface of the body are called dermatomes (refer to dermatome chart, page 21). Myotones are areas or groups of muscles which are innervated.

6. The thalamus, hypothalamus and pituitary gland are located at the base and center of the cerebrum. Temperature control, thirst, hunger, aggression, libido and integration with the endocrine system originate from this area.

Normal Physiological Functioning

1. Neural pathways between the lobes of the brain and the peripheral nervous system cross to the opposite side (contralateral). For example, domiant motor activity, such as right-handedness, is primarily governed by the left side of the brain.

2. Cranial nerves do not cross to the opposite side (ipsilateral); therefore, pressure on a cranial nerve will produce symptoms on the same side of the body as the intracranial pathology.

3. Voluntary movement by skeletal muscles is governed by the sensory and motor pathways in the parietal lobes. These pathways connect the brain with the peripheral nervous system and skeletal muscles as impulses travel through the midbrain and pons. Impulse transmission may be disrupted when these pathways are involved, producing skeletomuscular manifestations on the opposite side of the body.

4. Optimal metabolic activity of brain tissue requires an adequate and constant supply of oxygen and glucose. Therefore, 20% of each heart beat or cardiac output is delivered to the brain. Any disruption of cerebral circulation may lead to ischemia, hypoxia and cell death.

5. A balance is maintained between brain volume, blood and spinal fluid by changes in blood vessel size and CSF production. However, sudden increases in the volume of any of these three components, larger than 5-6 ml, will result in increased pressure and impaired cellular function.

Variations Related to Aging

1. Progressive visual and hearing impairment contribute to a feeling of isolation. A slower reaction time and impaired hearing can contribute to inappropriate responses and be interpreted as confusion or disorientation.

2. A decrease in brain fluid volume and increased adherence of meninges to the skull may result in injury to brain tissue after a minor fall.

3. The degeneration of intervertebral discs and osteoporosis leads to curvature of the spinal column with resulting restriction of chest movement and ventilatory capacity. This process also contributes to an increased incidence of compression vertebral fractures and subsequent pressure on spinal nerves.

4. The degeneration of sensory receptors of peripheral nerves contributes to an increased pain threshold. Early clinical manifestations of pathophysiological problems may be minimized or overlooked.

5. A decreased pumping capacity of the heart and atherosclerotic plaques may impair cerebral circulation.

6. Age-related changes in the function of the hypothalamus can lead to an altered sleep/wakefulness ratio and a decreased ability to regulate body temperature.

SECTION 2: INCREASED INTRACRANIAL PRESSURE (IICP)

Disrupted Physiological Functioning

1. Disruption of electrical impulse transmission within the brain results in a variety of patterns of symptoms (tremors, seizures, convulsions).

2. Minor changes in brain tissue, intracranial blood volume or CSF quickly impinge upon cerebral blood flow with resulting increased intracranial pressure. Cerebral capillaries become damaged secondary to impaired supply of oxygenated blood. The blood brain barrier which protects brain tissue from potentially harmful substances is altered. Fluid escapes from cerebral capillaries into the interstitial space (cerebral edema), further adding to the intracranial pressure.

3. A characteristic pattern of progression of intracranial pressure is detectable by nursing assessment. The level of responsiveness/consciousness is the most important and subtle indicator of a change in an intracranial condition.

Terms descriptive of altered states of consciousness:

* Conscious: Alert and responds appropriately to surroundings; body activities are controlled and coordinated; oriented to person, place and time. Situation or circumstance is often used for oriented X4.

* Confused: Awake and aware of surroundings but sometimes responds inaccurately/inappropriately.

* Disoriented: Awake but perceives surroundings and interactions inaccurately; responses are not related to the question asked.

* Obtunded: Reduced alertness; aroused by stimulation but quickly returns to a sleep-like state.

* Stuporous: Unresponsiveness; aroused only by vigorous and repeated stimuli; moans, opens eyes or withdraws from the source of stimulation.

* Comatose: Unarousable; protective reflexes such as eye blinking, coughing or gagging may remain intact.

Categories of irreversible brain damage:

* Persistent vegetative state: Chronically brain-damaged comatose state; vital signs including respirations are within normal limits (WNL); unaware and unresponsive to surroundings.

* Brain death: Physiological state in which there is no spontaneous respirations; no cerebral activity demonstrated on recordings of electrical impulse transmission recordings (EEG) or cerebral blood flow studies (angiography); cardiac and circulatory functions are reflex activities and are sustained by continuous medication.

Focused Neurological Assessment

Nursing assessment of the neurological status of high risk persons is crucial for the early detection and treatment of intracranial problems. Accuracy of assessment and prompt reporting of findings contribute to a favorable outcome.

Key symptoms suggestive of an adverse neurological change are:

* Restlessness with difficulty concentrating on personal activities

* Increasing difficulty awakening and staying awake

* Weakness or numbness, usually noticeable in the face with decreasing severity on one side of the body

Glasgow Coma Scale (GCS)

This standardized guide is widely used for assessing acute intracranial dysfunction and depth of coma. Numerical values are assigned to a person's BEST response for eye movements, verbal response and motor function.

Table 1-1. **Assessing Depth of Coma Using the Glasgow Coma Scale**

A total score is valuable in determining the severity of neurological damage. A score below 7 is comatose and is associated with severe damage and a poor prognosis.

Test	Score	Response
1. Best Verbal Response		
When you ask, "What day or year is this?" the person will respond with ...		
Oriented	5	Correctly names the day of the week or year.
Confused	4	States a name of the week or a year, but incorrectly.
Inappropriate	3	States something not related to the question asked.
Incomprehensible	2	Only moans or mumbles in response to tactile stimulus.
None	1	No response to painful stimulus.
2. Best Eye-Opening Response		
When you speak to this person, the response is ...		
Spontaneous	4	Opens eyes and looks at the speaker when spoken to.
To speech	3	Opens eyes after asked to do so.
To pain	2	Opens eyes only following painful stimulus.
None	1	No eye opening activity to any stimulus.
3. Best Motor Response		
When you ask the person to show you two fingers, the response is ...		
Obeys	6	Shows you the requested number of fingers using either hand.
Localizes	5	Reaches toward the source or location of the painful stimulus.
Withdraws	4	Moves away from the source or location of the painful stimulus.
Abnormal Flexion	3	Decorticate posture (below) in response to tactile or painful stimulus.
Abnormal Extension	2	Decerebrate posture (below) in response to tactile or painful stimulus.
None	1	No response; flaccid muscle tone.

Illustrations taken from L.A. Thelan, J.K. Davie, L.D. Urden, Textbook of Critical Care Nursing, 2nd ed.; St. Louis: Mosby-Year Book, Inc., 1994. Reprinted with permission.

Changes in Level of Consciousness (LOC)

1. Normally a person awakens easily and appropriately interacts with the surroundings by correctly responding to questions to determine orientation to person, place and time.

2. As intracranial changes occur, lethargy, drowsiness and difficulty arousing the person develop. Unexplained restlessness, irritability or forgetfulness are other characteristic findings.

3. The person is next asked to follow simple directions; such as blinking their eyes, moving an extremity or squeezing your hand.

4. If the person cannot respond to these directions, assessing the response to pain is the next step. Pinching and pricking soft tissue are avoided as bruising may occur. Nailbed pressure with a hard object (pencil or pen) normally elicits withdrawal from the source of pain. Vigorous rubbing on the sternum usually elicits eye opening in a comatose person.

5. If there is only minimal response to pain, assessing protective reflex activity is the next step. Spontaneous eyeblinking indicates the presence of the blink and corneal reflexes. Only if there is no blink response to stroking the eyelashes is it necessary to lightly touch the cornea with a sterile wisp of cotton.

6. If a person is able to speak, the gag reflex is present. Touching the posterior portion of the tongue may produce vomiting and unnecessarily increase the risk of aspiration.

7. Changes in the LOC are also the earliest signs of gradual healing of damaged tissue and the resolution of surrounding edema. Subtle indicators that the individual is more aware of their surroundings are detected by the nursing staff providing routine care. Several days or weeks may pass before signs of improvement are observable. Daily personal hygiene, linen change and communication provide a wide range of stimulating activities and the capability of responding.

Pupillary Responses

1. Pupils normally constrict to a light stimulus which is referred to as PEARL (pupils equal and react to light). To accurately elicit this response, the bedside should be dimly lit without the overhead lighting shining directly into a person's face. Penlight beam should be directed from the side of the face moving inward toward the eyes looking for pupillary constriction. The eyelids may need to be held open to determine the response.

2. As cranial nerves leave the brain stem directly, a change in pupillary response is consistent with hemisphere involvement (ipsilateral). For example, a sluggish response of the right pupil is associated with a lesion in the right side of the brain.

3. Increasing intracranial pressure on cranial nerve III causes a slowing or sluggish response. Fixed, dilated (unresponsive) pupil is an ominous sign of severe pressure.

Vital Sign Changes Accompanying IICP

1. The systolic blood pressure gradually rises causing a widening pulse pressure (the difference between systolic and diastolic BP).

2. A slow, bounding pulse rate accompanies the characteristic blood pressure changes. It is not unusual to observe a regular pulse rate below 60 beats per minute for a young adult following a head injury.

3. Changes in respiratory patterns occur with direct or indirect pressure on the respiratory center in the medulla. Supratentorial lesions or cerebral edema do not characteristically produce altered breathing until the condition is advanced. Whereas, infratentorial lesions may cause apneic episodes relatively early.

4. Difficulty maintaining the body temperature in the absence of an infection is another ominous sign. Pressure on the hypothalamus causes wide fluctuations in body temperature. An elevated body temperature increases the metabolic rate and oxygen needs of brain tissue which further compromises cerebral cellular functioning.

Alterations in Motor Function

1. Assessment of motor function is often accomplished while assessing the LOC. Movement and strength on both sides of the body (symmetry) is important for identifying the location of some intracranial lesions.

2. Unlike cranial nerves, motor pathways cross producing changes in movement and strength on the side of the body opposite of the hemisphere involvement. For example, weakness (paresis) or paralysis (plegia) on the left side of the body is associated with an intracranial lesion in the right side of the brain.

3. When deep coma is present and brain damage is severe, abnormal motor response (posturing) may occur. Posturing is a generalized and abnormal response to minimal tactile stimulation or movement of the person's immediate surroundings with the legs in rigid extension and the upper extremities flexed or extended.

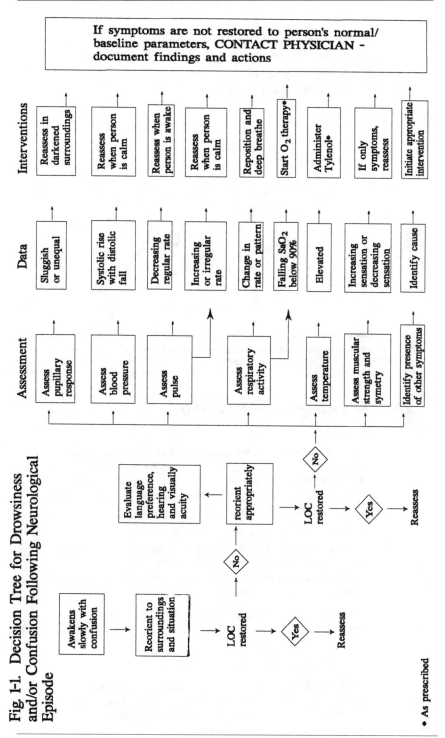

Fig 1-1. Decision Tree for Drowsiness and/or Confusion Following Neurological Episode

* As prescribed

4. Decorticate response includes spastic flexion of the arms, wrists and hands toward the midline of the body (adduction flexion).

5. Decerebrate response includes extensor spasm of all extremities which indicates a grave prognosis.

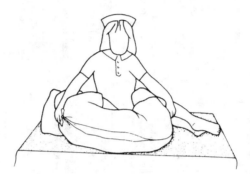

Fig. 1-2. Lumbar puncture position. From A.G. Perry, P.A. Potter: *Clinical Nursing Skills and Techniques: Basic, Intermediate, and Advanced*, 3rd ed.; St. Louis: Mosby-Year Book, Inc., 1994. Reprinted with permission.

Common Diagnostic Procedures

1. Lumbar puncture

   — Cerebrospinal fluid samples are obtained by inserting a sterile needle into the subarachnoid space between the third and fourth lumbar vertebrae, below the level of the spinal cord. The fluid is analyzed for electrolytes, glucose, protein and cells and the pressure is measured.

   — As this procedure is usually done at the bedside, a nurse assists with the preparation of equipment and positioning the patient. Familiarity of the neurological status prior to the procedure is valuable when determining the patient's response during and after the procedure.

   — Encouraging the patient to remain flat in bed in a dimly lighted room for several hours after the procedure diminishes the possibility of a headache.

2. Computed Tomography (CT)

   — Sophisticated equipment and non-invasive procedures are now available to provide more information about intracranial conditions than conventional radiographic techniques.

- Computerized assisted tomography or CAT scan obtains a series of images from specific layers of the brain to detect abnormalities.

- Magnetic resonance imaging (MRI) is another method for scanning the brain using a very strong magnet, radio frequency waves and a computer.

3. Cerebral angiography (blood flow study)

- This procedure is the radiographic visualization of the cerebral arterial system using a dye that is injected into the carotid artery. The adequacy of blood flow, identification of vascular abnormalities and the location of space-occupying lesions can be determined.

4. Electroencephalogram (EEG)

- The transmission of electrical impulses of the brain are recorded on paper. Characteristic and abnormal patterns are identified.

Interventions for Optimal Cerebral Functioning

1. Optimal cerebral function is dependent upon optimal cerebral blood flow. Several neurological factors as well as the adequate functioning of the heart and lungs are important. Sufficient amounts of oxygen must be inhaled and transported into the blood. Adequate quantities of hemoglobin and red blood cells must be in circulation to carry the oxygen to the brain. The pumping capacity of the heart must deliver a sufficient volume of oxygenated blood to the brain. Without this cardiopulmonary support, a relatively minor intracranial condition will become a serious problem due to the resulting cerebral hypoxia.

2. The neck is maintained in the midline position without flexion, extension or lateral rotation. Non-midline positions may interfere with arterial blood flow to the brain or venous return.

3. 15-30 degree elevation of the head of the bed is usually preferred over flat or high elevation. Venous return is facilitated with a slight head-of-the-bed elevation.

4. The use of a pillow under the head is avoided as it usually causes neck flexion.

5. Supplemental oxygen is usually administered prior to procedures for clearing the airway. Sustained coughing or suctioning longer than 15 seconds may deplete the oxygen supply to the brain.

6. Maintaining an adequate airway and clear pulmonary system is basic to adequate cerebral oxygenation.

Seizure Precautions

The risk for seizure activity is increased with disrupted physiological function due to a supratentorial lesion, such as cerebral brain tumor, cerebral vascular accident, ruptured cerebral blood vessel, meningitis, encephalitis, cerebral hematomas, cerebral head injuries. The risk is markedly decreased when the etiology is located below the tentorium.

1. Abnormal impulse transmission within the CNS due to supraten-torial lesions causes characteristic patterns of skeletal muscle responses. The tonic phase refers to profound muscle contraction. The clonic phase refers to alternating muscle contraction and relaxation. The term absence is preferred over the term petit mal, and clonic, tonic, or tonic-clonic are preferred over grand mal.

2. The pattern may be localized (tremor or twitch) or vigorous, generalized (grand mal). Documentation of the pattern should be accurately recorded which serves as a baseline as well as identifies any deviations from an established pattern.

3. If consciousness is lost, airway problems may develop due to obstruction of the tongue or aspiration of secretions. Placing the person on their side will allow secretions to drain from the mouth. In this position the tongue will not obstruct the airway. Bladder and/or bowel control may be lost.

4. After a grand mal seizure (postictal state), persons may be confused and very tired.

5. Restraint of extremities may cause injury to soft tissue or bones.

6. An oral airway or rolled washcloth may minimize tongue injury and maintain a patent airway. The use of other objects, such as a pencil or tongue blade is avoided as they may be broken by the strong muscle contractions of the jaw.

7. Prophylactic anticonvulsant medication is prescribed to minimize occurrence and severity of seizure activity. Tegretole (carbamazepine), Depakene (valproic acid) and Zarontin (ethosuximide) are recent medications for generalized seizures. Ativan is recommended for the treatment of status epilepticus. Conscientious oral hygiene prevents gingivitis and dental disease frequently seen with long-term Dilantin therapy.

8. Prolonged and/or continuous seizure activity is called status epilepticus and is regarded as an emergency situation as it can result in secondary brain damage due to cerebral hypoxia.

Care of an Unconscious Person

1. Conscientious, meticulous and on-going nursing care determines long-term outcomes and prevents disuse complications.

2. Nutritional support by hyperalimentation is provided until adequate peristaltic activity returns. Long-term enteral feedings may be required (nasogastric tube or gastrostomy).

3. Automatic urinary bladder emptying is difficult to manage. External or indwelling catheters present risk for infection or skin breakdown.

4. Routine bowel elimination or evacuation is essential to prevent constipation and fecal impaction.

5. Pre-menopausal women will resume monthly menstrual activity when the unconscious state is stable.

6. Diminished blink reflex and tearing may require the instillation of artificial tears inside the lower eyelid to prevent corneal damage.

7. Decreased secretions and mouth breathing leads to oral mucosa drying and tissue damage.

Meaningful Stimulation

1. Due to limited response by an unconscious person, care providers can easily become focused on body functions to the exclusion of psychosocial factors.

2. Meaningful stimulation is incorporated into the care regime as soon as the intracranial status is stabilized. An optimal 24-hour schedule includes sleep and wake cycles which resemble the person's pre-incident lifestyle.

3. Hearing is a strong sense that remains functioning even when no apparent response is observed. Conversations at the bedside should include the person as if hearing is intact. Address the person with respect and avoid informal names, such as "gramps" or "sweetie." Discussions about poor diagnosis, other patients or personal topics are best conducted beyond the patient's hearing range.

4. Tapes of family conversations or favorite music can be played intermittently by cassette player with earphones. Music may block environmental noise and promote restful sleep. Tapes of family interactions may stimulate consciousness when used after personal care activities when the patient is most aroused and capable of hearing and responding.

5. Touch, such as soothing stroking of an arm or holding a hand, is a medium for communicating caring and should be encouraged. Family may welcome the opportunity to participate in personal care such as hair combing, providing a backrub or foot massage.

6. To avoid startling the person, speak before touching and always introduce self with a brief, concise orientation to day and time.

7. As consciousness is regained, the response to stimulation may change, and a person may become agitated rather than soothed. The person may be confused with multiple stimuli which may agitate and escalate confusion. A calm, quiet and unhurried manner using a low-tone voice is usually stabilizing.

8. Avoid treating the confused adult as a child or incapable person. Positive reinforcement of accomplishments, even the smallest success, strengthens repeated positive and desired performance.

SECTION 3: EXAMPLES OF COMMON INTRACRANIAL CONDITIONS

Brain Tumors

Intracranial tumors may be benign, malignant or metastatic. All are space-occupying lesions which increase the volume within the skull and compress the surrounding brain tissue. Persons with suspected brain tumors may be hospitalized in a general medical-surgical unit prior to surgery. During this time, assessment of their neurological status is important as it will serve as a baseline for comparison during the immediate post-operative and convalescent periods.

1. These persons are at risk for seizures especially if the lesion is supratentorial. Risk for falling accidents is also increased due to possible unstable coordination. Establishing a safe environment is important.

2. Headaches, especially upon rising in the morning or at onset of seizure activity, are the most common manifestations observed in adults with brain tumors.

3. The immediate post-operative period is usually in the intensive care unit until the neurological status is stabilized.

4. A large head dressing is present and some portion of the hair has been removed.

5. Periorbital swelling usually occurs within 24-48 hours after surgery and may last several days. Cool compresses on the eyelids are soothing. The degree of edema may interfere with pupillary assessment.

6. Interventions to promote optimal cerebral functioning and meaningful stimulation are important. The process of healing and restoration of neurological function within the closed compartment of the skull is slower than the healing of other body tissues. Regeneration of neural tissue is only possible for those pathways protected by the myelin sheath. Other neural tissue will scar resulting in permanent disrupted function. It often takes weeks to determine the extent of permanent damage (neurological deficit).

Cerebral Vascular Accident (CVA or stroke)

This is the most common intracranial condition affecting adults. It is due to: (a) thrombosis or blood clot obstructing a cerebral artery; (b) rupture of a cerebral artery causing a cerebral hemorrhage; or (c) an embolus, fragment of a blood clot or atherosclerotic plaque, which traveled from the left side of the heart or carotid artery to a smaller cerebral artery. An underlying atherosclerotic condition is usually present. The management of the associated hypertension or plaque formation in larger vessels is a major preventive approach. Carotid endarterectomy procedure removes placque formation to improve the blood supply to the brain. The latest medical intervention for an acute CVA is thrombolytic therapy of occluded cerebral vessels.

1. Risk factors for developing a CVA: hypertension, diabetes mellitus, cigarette smoking, advancing age, Black ethnicity. At risk persons being treated for another physiological condition may concurrently develop an acute cerebral vascular problem. Neurological symptoms unrelated to the primary condition are essential to detect, such as sagging, weakened facial muscles, numbness, increasing difficulty awakening or staying awake or increasing restlessness with difficulty concentrating on personal activities.

2. Transient ischemic attack (TIA) is a brief episode of neurological deficit that passes without apparent residual effects. TIA is considered a warning signal of advancing atherosclerotic disease and impaired cerebral arterial supply.

3. Completed stroke refers to neurological deficit that remains unchanged over a 2-3 day period, whereas an evolving stroke refers to the progressive development of neurological symptomology.

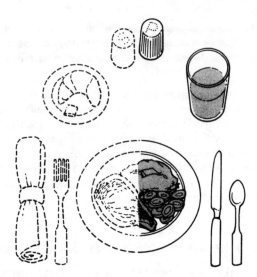

Fig. 1-3. Spatial/perceptual deficits in stroke. From S.M. Lewis, I.C. Collier: Medical Surgical-Nursing: Assessment and Management of Clinical Problems, 4th ed.; St. Louis: Mosby-Year Book, Inc., 1995. Reprinted with permission.

4.   Following a CVA due to a blood clot in a cerebral artery, anti-coagulant therapy (Heparin or Coumadin) may be used to minimize the extension of the blood clot. This medication classification does not remove or dissolve an existing clot; it minimizes clot formation. The dosage is determined by either a prothrombin time (PT) or partial thromboplastin time (PTT).

5.   Persons with dominant (left) hemisphere involvement have right-sided weakness or paralysis. Speech-language deficits are present, accompanied by distress and depression in relation to their disability. Their behavior style is slow and cautious. They need frequent reminders about their environment and once familiar objects.

6.   Persons with nondominant (right) hemisphere involvement are typically unaware of diminished abilities. They tend to be impulsive and have impaired judgment about their surroundings and therefore are at risk for injury.

7.   The loss of sensation of one side of the body alters the perception of the center of the body. Maintaining upright sitting and standing positions often need to be relearned. The location of pieces of furniture or doorway openings are distorted, increasing the likelihood of impact accidents. Similarly, blindness of half of the visual field accounts for inattention to objects not seen, such that food on one side is not seen and thus not eaten.

8. Flexor muscles usually retain strength longer than extensor muscles. Therefore, if preventive intervention is not consistently implemented, joint stiffening in flexed positions occurs (contracture). Arms tend to move inward toward the center of the body with flexion of the elbow and wrist. Legs tend to rotate outward at the hip with flexion of the knee and foot (foot drop).

9. The weight of flaccid paralysis of an arm may overstretch the shoulder joint. Partial dislocation and severe pain may result. Pulling on an affected arm when turning a stroke person can aggravate the problem. Supporting the affected arm in a sling or with pillows decreases the possibility of shoulder injury. Placing the affected arm in the sleeve first when putting on a hospital gown or shirt minimizes twisting injury to the shoulder.

10. Persons with aphasia have varying forms of expression and/or receptive problems. They may be able to understand what is said to them but cannot respond appropriately or they may not be able to understand what is said and therefore respond inappropriately.

Head Injuries

Impact trauma to the head results in a variety of injuries to the brain with the potential for neurological dysfunction and deficit. A person with an acute, unstable head injury usually requires continuous monitoring. Often the person with altered consciousness may also require mechanical ventilation.

During convalescence, conscientious nursing care is required to prevent the complications of immobility. Assessment of the subtle changes of improved IICP and responsiveness are detected during bedside care. However, occasionally the intracranial status may deteriorate, the early detection of changes can avert an irreversible complication.

Terms descriptive of various intracranial trauma:

* Concussion is a sudden, transient disruption of neural activity and a change in LOC with or without loss of consciousness.

* Postconcussion syndrome is seen 2 weeks to 2 months following concussion. Symptoms include persistent, recurring headache, lethargy and short attention span.

* Contusion is a bruising of brain tissue that is usually located at the site of a skull fracture.

* Epidural hematoma is a rapidly developing blood clot from a small arteriole. Bleeding occurs above the dura mater (meninges) and requires immediate treatment.

* Subdural hematoma is a slower developing blood clot from a
   small venule below the dura mater. Symptoms often become apparent 2-14 days after injury.

1. Injury to meninges may occur with a skull fracture. Leaking of CSF
   may be observed from the nose or ear with basal skull fractures.
   CSF drainage on clean, white bed linen appears in rings with the
   outer edges clearer than the inner portion, a halo appearance.
   There is increased risk for ascending infection and development
   of meningitis or encephalitis.

2. Accurate assessment of neurological function is crucial as IICP
   may develop. Examining assessment data for trends or patterns
   will detect subtle improvement or deterioration of the intracranial
   injury.

3. Symptoms of brain injury in the elderly often mimic other health
   problems. They may be overlooked resulting in a delay of treatment.

4. Optimal cerebral functioning and meaningful stimulation are collaborative interventions planned and implemented between
   nurses and physicians.

Meningitis

CNS infections may enter from the bloodstream or by extension from
a penetrating trauma. When the infection involves the coverings of
the brain, it is called meningitis. When the brain tissue is infected, it is
called encephalitis. If the infection is localized within the brain tissue,
it is called a brain abscess. This latter type of infection is often a result of embolic fragments from infectious colonies originating in the left
ventricles of the heart (bacterial endocarditis).

1. Bacterial meningitis is the most common type and is a medical
   emergency as it has a high mortality rate.

2. Symptoms include: fever, severe headache and nuchal rigidity (stiff
   neck), IICP and seizures.

3. Examination of the CSF obtained by lumbar puncture confirms the
   diagnosis. CSF protein levels are elevated. CSF glucose is decreased. CSF pressure is elevated and the fluid appears cloudy.

4. Swelling of the meninges and the potential for scarring may interfere with the reabsorption of CSF. An excess accumulation of
   CSF within the subarachnoid space and ventricles may occur (acquired hydrocephalus).

5. The blood-brain barrier normally protects brain tissue from potentially harmful substances. This protection mechanism, however, inhibits the effectiveness of many antibiotics. Only a few antibiotics penetrate the barrier: penicillin, ampicillin, chloramphenicol, nafcillin. During an acute neurological infection, these medications are administered in relatively high doses evenly-divided over each 24-hour period. Intrathecal administration of antibiotics may be necessary to achieve therapeutic outcomes. With this method, medication is introduced into the spinal fluid of the subarachnoid space.

Cerebral Aneurysm and Subarachnoid Hemorrhage

An aneurysm is a bulging of a cerebral artery. It is usually located at the base of the brain and is asymptomatic until it bleeds or ruptures. While the resultant cerebral hemorrhage may involve only a few ml of blood, the damage to neural tissue and subsequent cerebral edema pressure causes a life-threatening clinical situation.

1. Sudden onset of a severe headache quickly results in unconsciousness and rapidly progressing IICP.

2. Initially, continuous bedside monitoring of the intracranial status is required. The depth of consciousness may require mechanical ventilation. Therefore, care is provided in an intensive care unit.

3. When bleeding is stabilized, surgical ligation of the involved vessel is performed. Following post-operative and intracranial stabilization, the patient recovers slowly similar to the pattern of other intracranial neurological conditions. Several weeks may pass before the degree of neurological deficit can be determined.

SECTION 4: SPINAL CORD DYSFUNCTION

Persons with normal (intact) sensation and motor function of central neural pathways and the peripheral nervous system are aware of their body and able to voluntarily move body parts as the need and desire arises. However, when a person has impaired neural pathways in the brain, such as a contusion of the pons, the sensory and/or motor impulse transmission between the brain and skeletal muscles is disrupted. Trauma or tumor of the spinal cord causes a similar disruption of impulse transmission at or below the level of involvement. When an injury is localized to selected vertebrae, the symptoms are specific to the spinal nerve affected. While the degree of dysfunction varies, the clinical symptoms are similar.

Disrupted Physiological Dysfunction

1. Pressure, damage or severing of neural tissue interferes with impulse transmission along the pathway. The symptoms are specific to the level of spinal cord or spinal nerve involved. By accurate assessment of clinical manifestations, the location of involved dysfunction can be identified.

2. Some pathways transmit impulses from skeletal muscles or body parts to the brain (afferent/sensory pathways). Numbness, tingling and loss of sensation (paraesthesia) are associated symptoms.

3. Other pathways transmit impulses to skeletal muscles or body parts from the brain (efferent/motor pathways). Weakness (paresis) and paralysis (plegia) are associated symptoms.

4. Injury to the spinal cord or spinal nerves is usually secondary to injury to the vertebral column. The bony structures are compressed, rotated, hyperflexed or hyperextended to the point that a dislocation or fracture occurs.

5. Neural tissue is compressed, pulled, sheared or severed. Remember that neural tissue does not regenerate; it scars as it heals. Impulse transmission is disrupted or distorted.

6. If the damage is complete, such as a transection of the spinal cord, the continuity of sensory and motor impulse transmission is permanently disrupted and normal activity at or below the level of injury ceases.

7. Oftentimes inflammatory edema secondary to the trauma causes temporary loss of function. After the edema subsides, permanent neurological deficit can be determined.

8. Traumatic injury to the vertebral column may cause compression to the cushion-like intervertebral disc and the center portion of the disc will protrude or herniate. This response is like stepping on an ice cream sandwich and the inside squeezes out. The protruded portion of the disc causes pressure on a specific spinal nerve. Refer to the dermatome chart (below) to identify sensory or motor symptoms.

9. Degenerative changes of the disc gradually occur with aging and often result in a flexion curvature of the spine (kyphosis). When osteoporosis, a degenerative change in the bone, is also present, a fracture of thoracic vertebrae and compression of the intervertebral disc with pressure on specific spinal nerves may result.

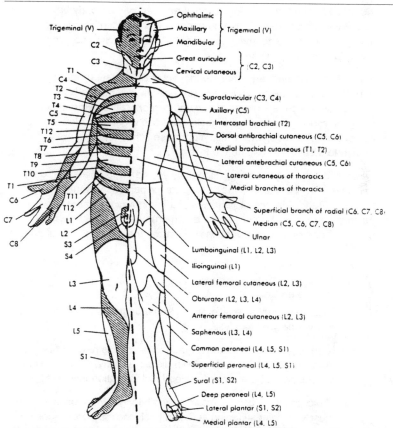

Fig. 1-4. Peripheral distribution of sensory nerve fibers (anterior view). Right, distribution of cutaneous nerves. Left, dermatomes (shaded) or segmental distribution of cutaneous nerves. From W.J. Phipps, B.C. Long, N.F. Woods: _Medical-Surgical Nursing: Concepts and Clinical Practices_, 5th Ed; St. Louis: Mosby-Year Book, Inc. 1995. Reprinted with permission.

Implications of Peripheral Neurological Dysfunction

To appreciate the impact of sensory and motor loss experienced by a person with quadriplegia, participate in the following mental exercise.

As you sit in a chair reading this book, concentrate only on the tactile sensations involving the right side of your body as it touches the chair that you are sitting on. Close your eyes and feel how the center of your body shifts. Be aware of the sensation that you are either moving to the left side with "feeling" or to the right side that has "no feeling." Hopefully it is easier to appreciate how difficult it is for a person with hemiparesis and hemiplegia to maintain an upright position. Balance becomes a conscious effort and often must be relearned.

Continue with a similar mental exercise. As you sit in this chair, imagine that you can feel but cannot move any part of your body below your waist (paraparesis). As you become tired of sitting in one position, you are unable to shift your weight. Your buttocks and thighs begin to hurt, but you cannot move.

Now close your eyes and imagine that you can not feel or move any part of your body below your waist (paraplegia). Allow the level of loss to rise to your shoulders. Now you can only shrug your shoulders and move your head and neck. You can wiggle your left little finger but cannot move your arms. Your nose itches and you are unable to scratch it. Imagine the frustration.

Relax and scratch your nose. Hopefully you can appreciate that daily self-care activities become major projects for persons with neural dysfunction. As the degree of paralysis and immobility increases, optimal functioning of other body systems is compromised. The implementations of appropriate interventions minimizes the development of complications.

1. General considerations
    — Decrease in muscle size and strength begins within three days of immobility or paralysis.

    — Normally, muscle movement facilitates venous return of blood from the legs to the heart. With disuse atrophy, venous circulation slows, and the risk for blood clot formation increases.

    — Flexor muscles usually retain strength longer than extensor muscles. Joint stiffening in flexed positions may occur (contracture). Arms tend to move inward toward the center of the body with flexion of the elbow and wrist. Legs tend to rotate outward at the hip with flexion of the knee and foot ("foot drop").

- Bone structure is maintained by muscle movement and weight bearing activity. With disuse, the normal process of bone metabolism is altered and calcium is not replaced or is lost from long bones. Bones become porous (osteoporosis) and susceptible to breaking with minimal stress (pathological fractures).

2. Paralysis of one side of the body (hemiplegia)

   - Person can only feel and move the unaffected side of their body.

   - The center of gravity shifts toward the side with feeling (unaffected) or to the side with no feeling (affected). Maintaining balance becomes a conscious effort and often must be relearned. There is an increased risk for falling accidents.

3. Paralysis of lower extremities (paraplegia)

   - Person can only feel and move above the level of injury, usually the waist.

   - Due to the relaxation of abdominal muscles, forcible coughing to expel secretions may be impaired as well as voluntarily bearing down to facilitate defecation.

   - The loss of lower spinal nerve activity interferes with the sensation of a full urinary bladder and need to defecate. Control of incontinence and retention are on-going problems. Self-catheterization is preferred when feasible as it is associated with a decrease in UTI compared with permanent indwelling catheters.

   - Maintaining intact skin especially over bony prominences is another on-going preventive concern. For example, the pressure of tight-fitting shoes may cause skin damage before a paralyzed person recognizes the problem.

4. Paralysis of lower and upper extremities (quadriplegia)

   - Person can only feel and move above the level of injury, usually only the shoulder. Refer to the dermatome chart (page 21) for cervical involvement.

   - Intercostal muscles used for breathing are controlled by thoracic spinal nerves. Therefore, breathing is controlled primarily by the diaphragm which exits the spinal cord from the upper cervical vertebrae.

   - Forcible respiratory activity, such as coughing, removing respiratory secretions and sneezing are, difficult for many persons with quadriplegia because of the loss of intercostal muscular function. Stasis of secretions from a common cold may quickly lead to respiratory failure.

— Maintaining adequate urinary and intestinal elimination is individualized according to the person's physical abilities. Distention can produce a serious physiological response.

— Following complete loss of neural transmission, flaccid paralysis and paresthesia is present. Involuntary reflex responses develop later and cause spontaneous, uncontrolled flexion of some muscles.

Focused Bedside Assessment

The following data would be expected from a head-to-toe assessment of a stabilized peripheral neurological condition in which no other pathophysiological problem involving another body system is present.

* **General appearance:** Within normal limits (WNL).

* **Level of consciousness:** Within normal limits (WNL).

* **Head and neck:** If a suspected cervical condition is present, immobilization in midline anatomical alignment is essential.

* **Respiratory status:** The level of sensory loss serves as a guide for intercostal muscle and respiratory involvement. For example, the higher the level of numbness, the greater the respiratory impairment. (Refer to Unit 3.)

* **Cardiac status:** Within normal limits unless there is accompanying pain and anxiety which may cause an increased heart rate.

* **Abdomen:** Decreased peristalsis and abdominal distention are common during early convalescence following a spinal cord injury or immediate postoperative spinal surgery. Relaxed abdominal muscles may result in a soft, protruding abdomen for persons with paraplegia or quadriplegia.

* **Urinary elimination:** Urinary retention with involuntary emptying occur with paraplegia and quadriplegia. Urine should be clear. Cloudy appearance may indicate a urinary tract infection (UTI). Characteristic signs, such as painful urination, may not be detected by paralyzed persons. Lower spinal nerve dysfunction may decrease the sensation of a full bladder or need to defecate.

* **Extremities:** Sensation and degree of motor function are related to the level of spinal involvement. Refer to dermatome chart (page 21). Assess the range of motion, anatomical alignment, intact skin especially over bony prominences. Interstitial edema of dependent extremities and paralyzed extremities is common. Assess the adequacy peripheral circulation (Unit 2).

* When the person is turned on their side, the nurse assesses for signs of skin pressure on the sacrum, both trochanters and heels.

* If additional data is observed, a more detailed assessment of the involved system is required. Additional areas of physiological dysfunction may be present and confound the present peripheral neurological problem.

Table 1-2. Motor and Sensory Impairment with Spinal Cord Injury

C1 to C4	"High quadriplegia." Only diaphragmatic breathing. Shallow cough ability. Total flaccid paraplegia loss of sensation below neck.
C5 to C8	"Low quadriplegia." Intercostal paralysis. Difficult coughing. Some movement of arms. Limited strength.
T1 to T6	"High paraplegia." Paralysis and loss of sensation midchest. No bladder or bowel control.
T7 to T12	"Low paraplegia." Paralysis and loss of sensation below the waist. No bladder or bowel control.
L1 to L5	Some paralysis in leg muscles. Bladder and bowel control problems. Some loss of sensation in legs and pelvis.
S1 to S5	Some intermittent bladder and bowel control problems. Some paralysis, muscle weakness and loss of sensation in feet and perineum.

Common Diagnostic Procedures

1. Electromyogram (EMG) assesses the electrical impulse transmission to skeletal muscles to determine if the symptoms are caused by a neurological or muscular problem.

2. Myelogram is radiographic procedure in which radiopaque dye is injected into the subarachnoid space and x-rays are taken to identify the spinal lesion.

3. CT scanning is also used.

Interventions to Prevent Complications

1. Prevention of vertebral column injuries

   - Immobilization and maintaining anatomical alignment of involved vertebrae minimizes further damage to the spinal cord or nerves. This stabilization is achieved by skeletal traction for fractured and dislocated vertebrae. External traction (Buck's, pelvic or halter) and collars or corsets stabilize disc injuries.

   - Work-related activities which require repeated lifting in a forward, bent and twisted position are likely to cause damage to the lumbar intervertebral discs.

   - Education in good body mechanics using the larger muscles of the thighs rather than the smaller vertebral muscles and lumbar corsets are recommended for persons with repeated lifting activities.

— Seat and shoulder belts and headrests in vehicles minimize whiplash injury of cervical discs.

2. Non-surgical interventions

   — Positioning in appropriate body alignment minimizes the development of flexion deformities or contractures. A firm-supporting mattress maintains vertebral alignment.

   — Logroll turning minimizes rotating or twisting an unstable vertebral column.

   — Due to loss of sensation and impaired mobility, the risk of skin breakdown is increased. Conscientious, planned preventive measures can minimize the occurrence. Devices to distribute body weight over bony prominences are effective, such as an overlay mattress for bedrest persons, frequent changes of body positions, adequate nutrition, clean and dry skin surfaces.

   — Range of motion (ROM) exercises of affected extremities maintains flexibility of joints and minimize flexion deformities (contractures). Active movement of unaffected muscles maintains muscle tone and strength.

   — An upright supportive board at the end of the mattress or high-top sneakers minimize flexion of the feet and shortened heel tendons (foot drop). Rolls of linen and sandbags minimize hip rotation.

   — A pillow or sling provides arm support for flaccid shoulder paralysis and minimize dislocation.

   — Anti-embolic hose promotes venous return by providing external support to weakened or paralyzed muscles in the lower extremities.

   — Abdominal thrusts (Heimlich Maneuver) may be implemented to assist person with coughing and expectoration of secretions.

3. Surgical interventions

   — Laminectomy involves the removal of the posterior segment of a vertebrae for the removal of the protruded intervertebral disc or a spinal cord tumor.

   — Discectomy involves only removal of the damaged disc.

   — Spinal fusion permanently stabilizes involved vertebrae by the placement of bony chips which allow the involved vertebrae to grow together. The iliac crest is a common donor site for the bony fragments.

— When stabilization of multiple vertebrae is required, small metal rods are attached along the outside of the affected vertebrae. This procedure is often preformed to provide a fixed, stable vertebral column for persons with a transected cervical spinal cord and quadriplegia.

SECTION 5: EXAMPLES OF COMMON VERTEBRAL AND SPINAL CORD CONDITIONS

Intervertebral Disc Conditions

Each vertebrae of the spinal column has four surfaces which articulates with the adjacent vertebrae. There are 23 cartilage structures (discs) between vertebrae which facilitate body movement. A compressing force of vertebrae or degenerative changes of the disc itself, may cause the center or nucleus of the disc to herniate through the disc capsule resulting in pressure on a spinal nerve root with subsequent symptoms specific to the involved nerve.

1. General considerations

   — Rest the involved vertebrae with local heat and external traction (Buck's, pelvic, or halter) to relieve the secondary muscle spasms.

   — Skeletal muscle relaxants are also helpful in minimizing the spasms and pain.

   — External supports such as corsets or collars provide anatomical alignment and support during the initial healing phase.

   — The terms herniated nucleus pulposus (HNP), herniated disc, or "slipped disc" refer to this pathophysiological involvement.

2. Back injury or lumbar disc involvement

   — The most common lumbar herniations occur at L3-4, L5 and L5-S1. Lifting heavy objects using a bent over position and back muscles is a common precipitating incident.

   — The predominant symptom is low back pain which may radiate in unilateral, characteristic patterns associated with the specific nerve involvement. When the pain radiates down the back of the thigh, it is commonly referred to as sciatica.

- One diagnostic assessment involves straight leg raising with the hip flexed and the knee extended which will produce sciatic pain. Pain, tingling or loss of sensation of specific toes is also characteristic.

3. Whiplash or cervical disc involvement

   - Hyperflexion and hyperextension of the head and neck from an impact motor vehicle accident (MVA) from the rear is the most common mechanism leading to disc problems involving cervical vertebrae.

   - The most common cervical disc herniations occur at C5-C6 and C6-C7.

   - The predominant symptoms include pain, numbness, tingling and loss of sensation from the neck to the shoulder and down the arm with characteristic finger involvement. Refer to the dermatome chart (page 21) for specific nerve innervation.

Spinal Cord Injury and Rehabilitation Principles

The majority of injuries are a result of impact accidents involving motor vehicles, falling, gunshot wounds and contact sports. These injuries are considered one of the most devastating physical and emotional disabilities to young adults. Skilled, persistent care involving a variety of nursing interventions is required to assist the individual to achieve their maximum level of independence without recurrent complications.

1. Injury to the spinal cord is due to flexion, rotation, extension, or compression of vertebrae. The degree of spinal cord involvement may be complete or incomplete (partial).

2. Complete damage results in irreversible loss of motor and sensory function below the level of lesion or injury. Flaccid paralysis is characteristic.

3. Incomplete damage results in mixed loss of voluntary activity. Small hemorrhagic areas and/or edema may produce more severe symptoms initially. Permanent neurological deficit can be determined after the resolution of edema.

4. The higher the level of injury, the greater possibility of spinal shock secondary to peripheral vasodilation, venous pooling and decreased cardiac output. Therefore, initially after injury, the person is usually cared for in an intensive care unit where systemic vital signs can be closely monitored.

— Spinal shock generally lasts 7 to 10 days.

— Muscle spasticity below the level of injury, reflex emptying of the urinary bladder and return of reflexes indicates the resolution of spinal shock.

NOTE: The return of reflex muscle activity below the level of injury does not necessarily indicate return of neurological function and can easily be misinterpreted.

Care must be given not to foster false hope.

Surgical intervention (decompression laminectomy) is directed at decompressing the spinal cord and minimizing progressive neurological deficit. Spinal fusion and the insertion of Harrington rods alongside the vertebral column stabilizes the vertebral column for quadriplegic persons.

7. Awareness of the extent of injury is coupled with a sense of overwhelming loss. Working through the grief is a difficult and lifelong process and described in terms of adjustment rather than acceptance. The nurse should expect a wide range of emotional responses.

8. Autonomic dysreflexia (hyperreflexia) is a massive cardiovascular reaction to visceral stimulation in persons with spinal cord injury above T7. The most common causes are distended urinary bladder or rectum. This condition may be life-threatening, producing initial symptoms of severe hypertension, blurred vision, throbbing headache, marked diaphoresis and bradycardia. Relief of the cause usually restores circulatory stability. Persistent symptoms are treated with an alpha-adrenergic blocker (Regitine) or vasodilator (Apresoline).

9. Sexual rehabilitation is a major issue as the majority of injuries involve young adult males. The presence of rectal sphincter tone is associated with the capability of reflex sexual function, usually of short duration. Generally there is a lack of perineal sensation. Orgasm and ejaculation are usually not possible for men with complete lesions. Spinal-cord-injured females of childbearing age usually remain fertile, capable of becoming pregnant and vaginal delivery.

10. The cause of premature death for the quadriplegic person is usually respiratory insufficiency and complications. Whereas, recurrent urinary tract infections and skin breakdown cause problems for the paraplegic person.

Spinal Cord Tumors

Primary spinal cord tumors are relatively rare, less than 1% of all neo-plasms. They tend to be slow-growing and produce progressive symp-toms of compression and displacement of the cord and nerves. Most spinal cord tumors are metatastic lesions from the bone, breast, lung, prostate or kidney.

1. Localized vertebral pain with radiation along associated nerve com-pression is the most common early symptom. Activity, sneezing, coughing or lying down aggravate the pain.

2. Later, coldness, numbness and tingling in an extremity indicate sensory involvement. Increasing motor weakness, clumsiness and spasticity are progressive.

3. Decompression laminectomy relieves the pressure of the tumor. Chemotherapy appropriate for the primary lesion often minimizes the symptoms and pain.

SECTION 6: EXAMPLES OF COMMON NEUROGENIC CONDITIONS

Multiple Sclerosis

This is a chronic, degenerative progressive disease of the central ner-vous system characterized by destruction of the myelin sheath which is the protective covering of certain nerve fibers. The cause is un-known and is one of the most disabling conditions of young adults be-tween the ages of 20-40 years of age. The interruption and distortion of impulse transmission result in a variety of symptoms.

1. The progression of the disease follows a pattern of recurrence and remission of symptoms.

2. Early symptoms include fatigue, weakness, numbness, difficulty with coordination and loss of balance. Visual disturbances are commonly reported, such as diplopia, nystagmus, blurred vision, patchy blindness.

3. Treatment plan focuses on management of symptoms. Goals in-clude promotion of physical mobility, avoidance of injury, achieve-ment of bladder and bowel continence, improved self-care and strengthening of coping mechanisms.

Parkinson's Disease

This is a progressive neurologic disorder affecting the brain centers that control and regulate physical movement. It is characterized by slowed movement, resting tremor and muscle stiffness due to depletion of dopamine levels in the basal ganglia. This condition is the second most common neurogenic condition of the elderly.

1. The characteristic body posture includes head bent forward, stooped forward with a shuffling and propulsive gait and loss of normal arm swing.

2. Facial expression is minimal with mask-like appearance.

3. The characteristic resting tremor is more noticeable in the forearm and hands. The thumb moves against the fingers in a repetitive motion as if rolling something.

4. Levodopa (L-dopa) is the most effective drug therapy to control symptoms. Other pharmacotherapeutic agents are prescribed in combination for management of clinical symptoms and side effects of L-dopa.

5. For selected individuals, surgical destruction of part of the thalamus (thalamotomy) relieves excessive muscle contractions.

Guillain-Barré Syndrome

This is a clinical syndrome of unknown cause involving peripheral and cranial nerves. In the majority of cases, a gastrointestinal or respiratory viral infection precedes the onset of symptoms. Initial clinical manifestations are numbness, tingling and weakness in the legs which usually progresses upward to the upper extremities and facial muscles. There usually is motor loss of function with intact sensation.

1. Most individuals have full recovery over several months but about 10% are left with residual disability.

2. This condition is a medical emergency as the symptoms develop rapidly and often cause respiratory difficulty that may require mechanical ventilation.

3. Muscle atony may cause hypotension and sometimes necessitates the use of vasopressor agents to stabilize blood pressure to normal limits.

4. After stabilization of acute symptoms, the prolonged convalescence requires consistent management of care to prevent the complications associated with immobility.

5. Interventions to prevent complications secondary to immobility, such as urinary tract infections secondary to indwelling catheters, physiotherapy and ROM, and nutritional needs are essential.

unit 2

NURSING CARE OF ADULTS WITH

Respiratory Conditions

T*his unit addresses a wide variety of common recurring respiratory conditions of adults which result in some degree of impaired gas exchange and are cared for on general medical-surgical nursing units. The management and care of critical and unstable conditions which require individualized "high tech" monitoring and equipment, such as respiratory failure, acute respiratory distress syndrome (ARDS) and penetrating chest trauma, are not included. The care of an individual requiring mechanical ventilation also is not addressed.*

However, some persons on a general medical-surgical nursing unit are at risk for developing an acute respiratory episode. It is important for the non-critical care nurse to recognize impending respiratory failure. The recognition of the signs and symptoms of altered gas exchange and early initiation of interventions minimize the development of a respiratory crisis.

SECTION 1: OVERVIEW

The nursing care of adults with respiratory dysfunction encompasses a wide variety of pathophysiological conditions. Effective plans for care are based upon an understanding of the normal functioning of the pulmonary system.

Anatomical Considerations

1. The pulmonary system is made up of two lungs, conducting airways, pulmonary blood vessels and the chest wall or thoracic cage. The lungs are divided into lobes and each lobe is divided into segments. The space between the lungs which contains the heart is called the mediastinum.

2. A set of tubes or conducting airways permit the flow of air into each lung. The upper airway includes the nasal and oral pharynx. These structures are lined with ciliated mucosa which have a rich capillary blood supply. This lining warms and humidifies the air and removes foreign particles.

3. The larynx connects the upper and lower airways. The cartilaginous structures include the vocal cords and supporting rings which maintain the patency of the airway. The movable fold of tissue which covers or closes the opening of the airway during swallowing is called the epiglottis.

4. The structures below the larynx make up the lower airway. The trachea is the first and largest portion of the lower airway. Inside the thorax, the trachea divides into two bronchi which provide air flow into each lung. The smallest conducting airways are the bronchioles. The structures of the lower airway are also lined with mucous-secreting and ciliated cells.

5. The conducting airways lead into the gas exchange units: alveolar ducts, alveoli and pulmonary capillaries. A lipoprotein (surfactant) coats the inner surface of the alveoli to maintain expansion during inspiration and expiration. Approximately 25 million alveoli are present at birth and 300 million in healthy adult lungs.

6. The lungs are protected by a bony rib cage or the thorax. The movement of the muscles between the ribs (intercostal) and the diaphragm permit an adequate flow of air through the passages. Two layers of serous membrane cover the surface of the lungs. Normally only a thin layer of fluid is present between these layers for lubrication of the surfaces during respiratory activity. Pressure within the pleural space is negative and allows for maximum lung expansion.

Mechanics of Breathing

The physiological actions of the pulmonary system include ventilation (breathing) and gas exchange. Diffusion refers to the movement of gases between the air spaces in the lungs and the bloodstream. Perfusion is the transportation of gases throughout the circulatory system and is dependent upon the adequate functioning of the heart, vessels and red blood cells. Cardiopulmonary function refers to the close interrelationship between the two body systems. Understanding the components of breathing provides the rationale for optimal care of adults with an ineffective airway and/or impaired gas exchange nursing diagnoses.

1. Ventilation or breathing

   — This is a process of providing a constant air supply to the lungs. It includes the actions of inspiration (inhalation) and expiration (exhalation). Patent passages from the nose and mouth to the alveolar sacs are essential for optimal air movement.

   — The movement of the thoracic bones (ribs and clavicle), intercostal muscles and diaphragm change the pressure within the chest and influence the volume of air moved during each breath.

   — Normally, the muscular effort required for breathing is very low. However, when there is increased resistance to the airflow or increased oxygen requirements by the tissues, the workload can be markedly increased.

2. Air flow

   — As the diaphragm contracts, it lowers and thereby decreases the intrathoracic pressure. And, as the intercostal muscles raise the ribs, the chest enlarges. The pressure within the thorax and lung spaces decreases allowing atmospheric air to flow in through the passages to the alveoli (inhalation).

   — When the diaphragm relaxes, it moves upward and the air moves passively out of the lung (exhalation).

   — The capacity of the lungs to inhale and exhale (pulmonary function) is measured by an inspirometer and pulmonary function studies. An estimate of volume exchanged with a normal breath which is appropriate for body size (tidal volume/TV) is calculated by body weight (BW) in kilograms (Kg) multiplied by 8-10cc (TV = BW in Kg x 8-10cc).

3. Stimulus for respiratory activity
   — The primary stimulus to the respiratory center in the medulla oblongata and pons is a change in the amount of circulating carbon dioxide. As carbon dioxide levels increase ($paCO_2$ > 45 mmHg) respiratory activity increases.

   — Decreased oxygen levels in circulation (paO_2 <75-80 mmHg) is the secondary stimulus. Hypoxemia triggers increased respiratory activity when the primary stimulus is ineffective.

   — Chemoreceptors primarily located within the vascular and cerebospinal fluid systems and articular joints detect changes in the pH and circulating oxygen and carbon dioxide levels. These changes alter the rate and depth of respiratory activity.

Gas Exchange Cycle

The cycle of gas exchange begins at the alveolar sacs. It includes three components: (1) the inspiratory phase or oxygen delivery, (2) tissue/cellular oxygen consumption and metabolism, and (3) the expiratory phase or return of metabolic wastes such as carbon dioxide and unused oxygen.

With an understanding of the gas exchange cycle, one can appreciate the clinical context. There is overlap between ventilation and gas exchange as well as between inspiratory and expiratory problems. Often as inspiratory conditions become more serious, expiratory symptoms are observed. By the time many persons seek medical assistance, both inspiratory and expiratory symptoms are present. By recognizing the underlying problem and the sequence of developing pathophysiology, an astute nurse can determine the early signs of a worsening or improving clinical situation. Appropriate nursing actions can then be initiated.

1. Inspiratory phase (alveolar level)
   — Oxygen moves into the pulmonary capillaries. If an insufficient amount of inspired air reaches the alveoli, the amount of oxygen exchanged may be below normal (paO_2 < 75-80 mmHg) leading to hypoxemia.

   — Oxygenated blood moves through the pulmonary veins to the left side of the heart. From the left ventricle, the oxygenated blood is pumped into circulation through the aorta. Oxygen is transported to the periphery by way of the arteries.

Fig. 2-1. Gas Exchange Cycle

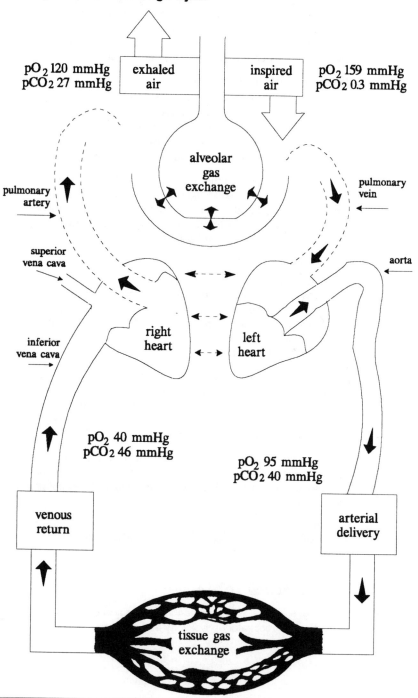

pO_2 120 mmHg
pCO_2 27 mmHg

exhaled air

inspired air

pO_2 159 mmHg
pCO_2 0.3 mmHg

alveolar gas exchange

pulmonary artery

pulmonary vein

superior vena cava

aorta

inferior vena cava

right heart

left heart

pO_2 40 mmHg
pCO_2 46 mmHg

pO_2 95 mmHg
pCO_2 40 mmHg

venous return

arterial delivery

tissue gas exchange

— Adequate perfusion or circulation of oxygenated blood is dependent upon an adequate hemoglobin level and an adequate number of erythrocytes. Efficient pumping capacity of the myocardium is essential for systemic perfusion which is reflected by a normal blood pressure and cardiac output.

2. Oxygen consumption (tissue level)

— At the periphery, oxygen leaves the capillary in sufficient amounts for aerobic cellular metabolism. If insufficient oxygen is available to the cells, tissue hypoxia and anaerobic metabolism occurs. An arterial oxygen saturation level (SaO_2) below 80% is associated with anaerobic cellular metabolism.

— The difference between the oxygen level in the arterial and venous circulation is an estimation of the oxygen utilization by the cells and is called oxygen consumption. When the cellular need for oxygen is greater than what can be delivered, an oxygen deficit exists and altered cellular metabolism occurs.

3. Expiratory phase

— The end product of aerobic cellular metabolism (carbon dioxide) passes into the capillaries and returns to the heart through veins. It enters the right side of the heart by way of the vena cava. From the right ventricle, blood returns to the lung through the pulmonary artery. Carbon dioxide moves into the alveoli and is exhaled.

— If the carbon dioxide is not able to move into the alveoli, it accumulates in the blood causing respiratory acidosis (hypercapnia). Conditions which may lead to this acid-base imbalance include markedly enlarged alveoli (emphysema), pulmonary embolus, fractured ribs or coma.

— The end products of anaerobic metabolism include lactic and pyruvic acids. These waste products also pass into the capillaries and are carried to the kidneys and eventually excreted in the urine.

  • An excess of lactic acid in the circulation is called lactic acidosis and is associated with a high mortality rate.

Variations Related to Aging

As a person ages, normal alterations and physiological changes occur which impact on the respiratory physiology and management of care.

1. As age advances, the alveoli tend to enlarge or atrophy with a progressive loss of capillary surfaces. As a result, there is a general decrease in the lung surface available for gas exchange.

    — The ribs become less flexible and stiffer, causing decreased chest expansion. Gradually the vital capacity decreases and the residual volume increases.

    — Elasticity of aveolar membranes decreases with decreasing ability of the lung tissue to expand and contract.

2. The chemoreceptors become less sensitive to circulating oxygen and carbon dioxide levels and the paO_2 values decrease proportionately with advancing years. It is not unusual to observe a paO_2 of 76 mmHg for an 80-year-old individual who has no apparent respiratory distress.

3. While there is a considerable difference among individuals, their activity, health status and general fitness, the elderly are less able to physiologically respond to gas exchange needs which accompany illness. For example, respiratory flu may quickly progress to pneumonia. Recovery is often slower and symptoms last longer.

4. Changes in vertebral alignment may produce a curvature (kyphosis) or compression fractures. These structural changes may decrease an elder's vital capacity and effective cough response.

5. The diaphragm, abdominal muscles and accessory muscles weaken with age, leading to progressively impaired exhalation.

SECTION 2: PULMONARY/ RESPIRATORY DYSFUNCTION

Overview

In recent years, significant changes have occurred in the incidence and prevalence of pulmonary conditions. Environmental and occupational lung diseases related to dust particles or pollution have steadily risen. Nosocomial and opportunistic pulmonary infections have increased the morbidity for immunosuppressed individuals. However, cigarette smoking is attributed to the development of the major pulmonary conditions: lung cancer and chronic obstructive pulmonary disease (COPD).

Assessment of Pulmonary/Respiratory Status

1. General appearance
   - An individual's ease in breathing can be easily assessed during an initial nursing contact. Does the individual appear comfortable and able to breathe without effort? Is the individual able to lie flat without respiratory distress or what position facilitates breathing? Does speaking affect the breathing pattern?

2. Respiratory rate and depth
   - The individual's baseline of respiratory rate and depth should be established and used for comparison when evaluating the person's tolerance to activity and response to therapeutic interventions. Baseline data may vary among individuals and their respiratory dysfunction. A change in the rate or depth of respirations may be within the normal expectations for one individual and unusual for another.

   - An absence of periodic sighing decreases the expansion of alveoli and may lead to the development of collapsed areas of lung tissue (atelectasis). Diminished sighing may occur during the immediate post-operative period and following heavy sedation.

   - Tachypnea refers to fast and shallow respirations. When this pattern occurs at rest, it is usually associated with an elevated body temperature, chest pain or hypoxemia.

   - Bradypnea refers to slow but regular respirations. When this pattern occurs, it is usually associated with increased intracranial pressure, heavy sedation or deep sleep.

   - Hyperventilation refers to increased rate and depth of respirations. It is an anticipated response to increased physical activity and may also occur with increased anxiety. As hyperventilation increases the exhalation of carbon dioxide, it can produce the sensation of lightheadedness and lead to fainting (syncope).

   - Kussmaul respirations describe a characteristic pattern of very deep respirations. This pattern is associated with a physiological response to exhale excess carbon dioxide or as an attempt to compensate for an underlying acidotic state. It is observed in states of metabolic acidosis and diabetic ketoacidosis (DKA).

   - Cheyne-Stokes respirations describe a characteristic cyclic pattern of deep respirations followed by progressively more shallow respirations with periods of apnea. This pattern is an ominous sign of brain damage.

3. Mental status

    — A change in an individual's mental status may be an indirect
       assessment of the adequacy of perfusion of oxygen and car-
       bon dioxide within the brain. A sensation of lightheadedness
       or fainting may indicate decreased carbon dioxide in the cere-
       bral circulation.

    — Indicators of cerebral hypoxemia (below normal levels of oxy-
       gen) include increased anxiety, restlessness, irritability and
       poor concentration. Indicators of cerebral hypercapnia (ele-
       vated levels of circulating carbon dioxide) include lethargy, con-
       fusion and sleepiness.

4. Skin color

    — Changes in skin color provide unreliable data when assessed
       in isolation. Many other structural, physiological and environ-
       mental factors influence changes in peripheral skin color.
       Therefore, when cyanosis is observed, additional data should
       be identified to determine to adequacy of respiratory function
       and gas exchange.

    — Lack of cyanosis does not necessarily indicate adequate oxy-
       genation. For example, anemia can cause inadequate tissue
       oxygenation without cyanosis.

    — With acute respiratory distress, the skin is often diaphoretic in
       addition to the presence of pallor or cyanosis.

5. Shortness of breath (dyspnea)

    — Dyspnea is a subjective sensation of breathlessness, short-
       ness of breath (SOB) or respiratory distress. Varying degrees
       of anxiety and preoccupation with breathing accompany dys-
       pnea.

    — As the severity of dyspnea is often underestimated by health
       care providers, self assessment can usually be provided by
       the individual. Indicating dyspneic severity on a 1 to 10 scale
       or marking a point on a vertical line provides corroborating
       data.

    — Differentiating between breathlessness at rest and breathless-
       ness with exertion is important. Persons are often not aware
       of their dyspnea. One differentiating clue occurs when these
       individuals are talking. Dyspneic persons frequently interrupt
       themselves in midsentence to take rapid, shallow breaths.

    — Orthopnea is a type of dyspnea which occurs when the individ-
       ual is lying flat and is relieved by sitting upright.

- Paroxysmal nocturnal dyspnea (PND) refers to dyspneic episodes which occur at night and is associated with left ventricular cardiac failure.

- As the workload of breathing increases, the use of accessory muscles becomes more apparent. Elevation of the chest is augmented by sternocleidomastoid, pectoralis and trapezii muscles. Intercostal or sternal retraction is not commonly observed in adults.

6. Cough

- The presence of coughing and the production of sputum is important and is a normal physiological response to remove excess secretions and foreign materials from the airways. Therefore, pattern of coughing and nature of the sputum produced are data related to the etiology of the respiratory dysfunction or an indicator of effectiveness of an intervention to improve respiratory function.

- Sputum (phlegm) is the substance expelled by coughing or clearing the air passages. The color and quantity of sputum are helpful in determining the cause of respiratory dysfunction.

   • Clear or colorless sputum is usually due to a noninfectious process and likely an allergic response.

   • Creamy yellow sputum is usually due to a staphylococcal infection.

   • Greenish sputum is usually due to a pseudomonas infection.

- Hemoptysis refers to the presence of blood in the sputum. This abnormal symptom is often due to increased pressure within the pulmonary capillaries (pulmonary hypertension).

- Epistaxis refers to a nosebleed and should not be confused with hemoptysis. Allergies, dry nasal mucosa or hypertension contribute to the occurrence and severity of epistaxes. Nasal packing applies pressure at the bleeding site. Sometimes cauterization of the bleeding vessel is required to stop the bleeding.

7. Chest pain

- Lung tissue has few neural receptors for pain. Therefore, some respiratory conditions can progress to a severe state before pain is felt by the individual. On the other hand, when the rib cage or pleura is involved, severe pain is characteristic at the onset of dysfunction.

- A sudden collapse of lung tissue which may occur with a spontaneous pneumothorax often produces sudden onset of sharp chest pain, marked dyspnea and hypoxia.

8. Lung sounds
   - The intensity and quality of breath sounds are heard by auscultation during inspiration and expiration. Bronchial sounds are normally heard over the larger air passages. Normal vesicular sounds are heard over the other lung fields during the respiratory cycle.
   - Adventitious sounds are not normally heard and are described as gurgles, wheezes, crackles, rhonchi and pleural friction rubs.
     - Crackles (rales) are described as interrupted bubbling or popping sounds originating from the smaller air passages.
     - Rhonchi are gurgling, snoring, continuous sounds caused by partially obstructed air passages.
     - Wheezes are high-pitched, continuous sounds associated with airway narrowing which are often more pronounced on expiration.
     - Stridor refers to high-pitched sounds audible during inspiration.
     - Pleural friction rubs are grating sounds associated with breathing when inflamed pleural surfaces move together.
   - Decreased breath sounds are identified over poorly aerated areas of lung tissue which may occur with atelectasis, obesity or shallow respiratory activity.
   - An absence of breath sounds may be associated with collapsed lung tissue which may occur with atelectasis or pneumothorax.

Arterial Blood Gas (ABG) Interpretation

The human body functions best in a state of homeostasis or balance. Sometimes physiological dysfunction disrupts this balance which may be reflected in an alteration in the acid-base balance. Considerable data gained from one ABG or a series of values increase the understanding of appropriate nursing action and medical management of individual clients.

In this unit, the changes in acid-base balance related to an underlying respiratory condition are presented. The body's mechanism to restore balance by the kidneys, which is referred to as metabolic compensation, are examined. Acid-base imbalances related to an underlying metabolic condition are discussed in Unit 6: Urinary Elimination Problems.

When interpreting a given ABG, these three steps should be followed:

1. First look at the pH.

    — Normal parameters (WNL) for pH are: 7.35-7.45.

    — If the pH of a given ABG is below 7.35, the acid-base imbalance is acidosis.

    — If the pH of a given ABG is above 7.45, the acid-base imbalance is alkalosis.

2. The second step determines the type of acid-base imbalance Look at the $paCO_2$ and HCO_3 values. At this time only those values associated with an underlying respiratory condition are presented.

    — Normal parameters (WNL) for $paCO_2$ are: 35-45 mmHg.

    — If the $paCO_2$ value is above 45 mmHg and the pH is below 7.35, then the primary acid-base imbalance is respiratory acidosis.

    — If the $paCO_2$ value is below 35 mmHg and the pH is above 7.45; then the primary acid-base imbalance is respiratory alkalosis.

    — With abnormal $paCO_2$ values and HCO_3 values WNL, the acid-base imbalance is called <u>UNCOMPENSATED</u> respira-tory acidosis or alkalosis. This is likely to occur with an acute respiratory condition as it usually takes 24-72 hours for the kidneys to respond by appropriately changing the HCO_3 levels.

    — If the $paCO_2$ value is WNL and the HCO_3 value is above or below normal parameters (22-26 mEq/L), then a metabolic imbalance is present. Conditions associated with primary metabolic acidosis or alkalosis are discussed in Unit 6: Urinary Elimination Problems.

3. The third step: Identify if compensation by the kidneys is present and to what extent. The HCO_3 value provides an indication of the kidneys' ability to balance the respiratory imbalance. The kidneys normally are able to generate or excrete bicarbonate ions and regulate the degree of excretion of hydrogen ions. The pH value will reflect the effectiveness of compensation to restore homeostasis.

    — Normal parameters (WNL) for HCO_3 are: 22-26 mEq/L.

    — When respiratory acidosis is present ($paCO_2$ above 45 mmHg), metabolic compensation will be reflected by a gradual rise in the HCO_3 value above normal parameter (26 mEq/L). The pH will also rise toward normal (7.35), but is not WNL.

— When respiratory alkalosis is present (paCO$_2$ below 35 mmHg), metabolic compensation will be reflected by a gradual decrease in the HCO$_3$ value below the normal parameter (< 22 mEq/L). The pH will decrease toward normal (7.45) but is not WNL. These acid-base imbalances are called <u>COMPEN-SATING</u> respiratory acidosis or alkalosis.

— When the metabolic compensation balances the respiratory imbalance, the pH will be WNL. A balance between a primary respiratory imbalance and metabolic compensation is called <u>COMPENSATED</u> respiratory acidosis or alkalosis.

Diagnostic Studies

1. Pulmonary function testing

   — A comprehensive assessment of respiratory capacity pro-vides valuable diagnostic data. The most frequently used data include the following:

   • Tidal volume (TV) refers to the volume of air moved in and out of the lungs during normal breathing activity.

   • Vital capacity (VC) refers to the maximum volume of air moved in and out of the lungs during forced breathing activity.

   • Residual volume (RV) refers to the amount of air remaining in the lungs after maximum expiration.

2. Chest x-rays

   — Chest films can be completed in the radiology department or at the bedside to visualize anatomical structures, intrathoracic equipment or air-filled lung tissue. Different densities pro-duce shades from white to grey or black on a film. Bone is very dense and appears white. Soft tissue, fluid and blood are less dense and appear as shades of grey. Air is the least dense and appears black.

   — Computerized techniques (CT scans, PET, MRI) provide more sophisticated visualization and can detect smaller lesions with greater accuracy.

3. Invasive procedures

   — Direct observation through a lighted scope of fiberoptic tubing may be performed to visualize the anatomical structures of the upper airway and major air passages. Laryngoscopy refers to the visualization of the larynx. Bronchoscopy refers to the visualization of the bronchi and may be done to remove a mucous plug from a bronchus.

If symptoms are not relieved or worsen following intervention,
CONTACT PHYSICIAN - document findings and actions

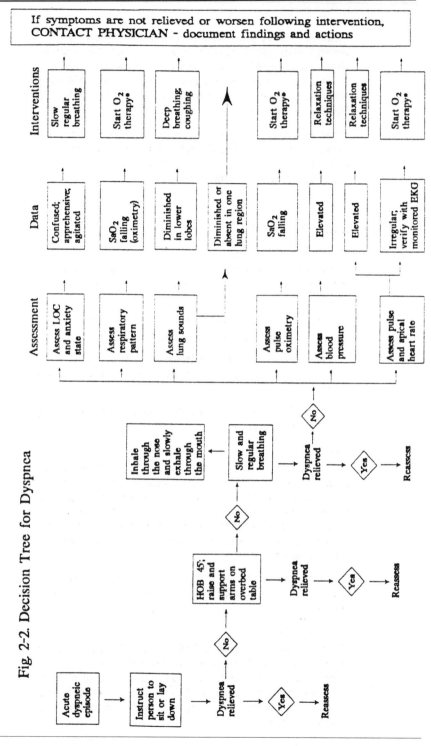

Fig 2-2. Decision Tree for Dyspnea

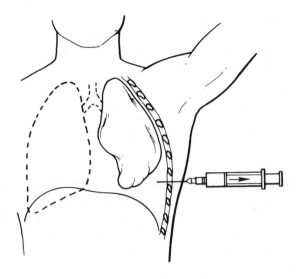

Fig. 2-3. Thoracentesis. *From S.M. Lewis, I.C. Collier: <u>Medical-Surgical Nursing: Assessment and Management of Clinical Problems</u>, 4th ed.; St. Louis: Mosby-Year Book, Inc., 1995. Reprinted with permission.*

    — Thoracentesis refers to the insertion of a sterile needle between the ribs into the pleural space to remove accumulated fluid. This procedure is usually done at the bedside. Usually less than 1200 cc is removed at one time to permit adequate lung re-expansion and physiological adaptation to the changes in inter-thoracic and circulatory pressures.

4. Sputum analysis

    — The mucous membrane of the respiratory tract responds to inflammation by an increased flow of secretions which often contain the causative infective organism. Obtaining a sputum specimen for culture and sensitivity (C&S) is done before antibiotics are started. The first sputum raised in the morning usually is most productive of organisms.

    — Acid-fast bacilli (AFB) testing determines the presence of the mycobacterium tuberculosis organism. Gastric washings may be required to locate the organism as many individuals frequently swallow their sputum.

5. Skin testing

— Testing for allergic hypersensitivity or exposure to specific organisms is not totally reliable and is not used as a sole basis for diagnosis. Sometimes recent illness, recent immunizations or some medications may produce false positive skin test results.

— PPD (purified protein derivative) or the tine test is used for screening to determine if an individual has been exposed to the tuberculosis bacillus. A positive response requires confirmation by x-ray and sputum analysis.

Measures to Improve Respiratory Efficiency

Independent and collaborative nursing interventions are initiated to intervene in the progression of pathophysiological events associated with respiratory dysfunction. The effectiveness of these interventions can minimize the development of complications.

1. Maintenance of a patent airway

— Chest physiotherapy (CPT) is a group of activities co-managed by nurses and respiratory therapists. When coughing is ineffective, additional measures are necessary to loosen sputum and clear the air passage, such as postural drainage, percussion and vibration.

— Suctioning the oral and air passages is co-managed by nurses and respiratory therapists. Tracheal suctioning is a sterile procedure for the removal of secretions from the tracheobronchial tree.

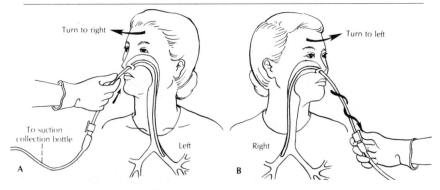

Fig. 2-4. Nasotracheal suctioning: Correct placement of suction catheter in (A) left and (B) right mainstream bronchi. From J. Luckmann, K.C. Sorensen: Chapter 30-Respiratory therapeutic intervention, Medical-Surgical Nursing: A Psychophysio-logic Approach, 4th ed. (D.Kay, Ed.); Philadelphia: W.B. Saunders Company, 1993. Reprinted with permission.

- To minimize the risk of hypoxemia and bradycardia, the administration of 100% oxygen is recommended before and following each pass of the suction catheter. Suctioning time should be limited to 15 seconds to minimize hypoxia.

- Suctioning oral secretions should follow tracheal suctioning to minimize contamination of air passages.

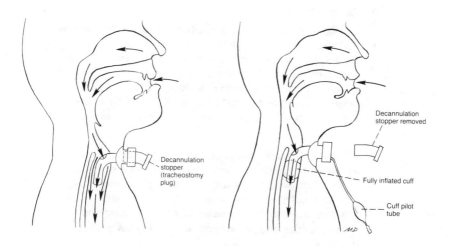

Fig. 2-5. Fenestrated tracheostomy tubes. From J. Luckmann, K.C. Sorensen: Chapter 32-Nursing people experiencing lower airway disorders, _Medical-Surgical Nursing: A Psychophisiologic Approach_, 4th ed. (D. Kay, Ed.); Philadelphia: W.B. Saunders Company, 1993. Reprinted with permission.

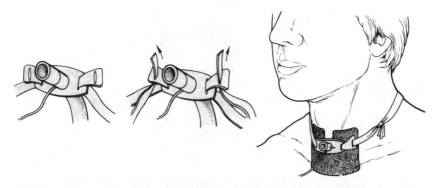

Fig. 2-6. Changing tracheostomy ties. From S.M. Lewis, I.C. Collier: _Medical-Surgical Nursing: Assessment Management of Clinical Problems_, 4th ed.; St. Louis: Mosby-Year Book, Inc., 1995. Reprinted with permission.

- A tracheostomy is an artificial opening in the trachea into which a metal or plastic tube is placed. The tube is secured by twill ties attached to each side of the tube. Once the operative opening is healed, the care is a clean procedure following universal precautions of the secretions. Speaking is possible when the opening is covered.

- A permanent tracheostomy is made following a total laryngectomy.

2. Breathing patterns
   - An incentive spirometer is a mechanical device that promotes sustained maximum inspiration and lung expansion. The person breathes in through the mouthpiece as deep as possible and holds the breath for at least 3 seconds. The ball or indicator raises within the chamber reflecting the volume of air inhaled. An optimal goal for deep breathing is 2 times the person's tidal volume or normal inspiratory and expiratory volume.

   - "Pursed-lip" and diaphragmatic breathing patterns are learned activities to increase the length and force of the expiratory phase of the ventilatory cycle. "Pursed-lip" breathing also maintains optimal airway pressure during exhalation. These activities increase the exhalation of carbon dioxide and minimize relaxation and possible collapse of the lower airway ducts.

     - "Smell the rose" during inhalation and "blow out a candle" during exhalation are helpful guides to teach diaphragmatic pursed lip breathing.

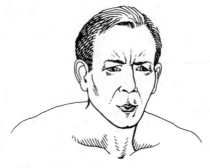

Fig. 2-7. Pursed-lip breathing. From W.J. Phipps, B.C. Long, N.F. Woods: <u>Medical-Surgical Nursing: Concepts and Clinical Practice</u>, 5th ed.; St. Louis: Mosby-Year Book, Inc., 1995. Reprinted with permission.

- Individuals prone to dyspnea need to learn how to conserve their oxygen consumption. The following resting positions are beneficial at the onset of a dyspneic episode.

  - Sitting forward in a chair with elbows supported (fig. 2-8, A).

  - Sitting and leaning over a stack of pillows or an overbed table with elbows supported (fig. 2-8, B).

  - Standing and leaning over the back of a chair (fig. 2-8, C).

  - Standing and leaning against the wall (fig. 2-8, D).

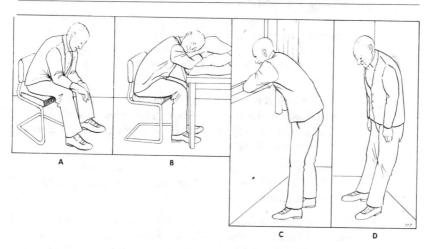

Fig. 2-8. **Dyspnea positions.** *From J. Luckmann, K.C. Sorensen: Chapter 30-Respiratory therapeutic intervention, Medical-Surgical Nursing: A Psychophysiologic Approach, 4th ed. (D. Kay, Ed.); Philadelphia: W.B. Saunders Company, 1993. Reprinted with permission.*

3. Oxygen therapy

   - On medical-surgical nursing units, humidified oxygen is usually administered by nasal cannula. The rate is between 1-4 Liters/minute and the flow (FiO2) is between 24-35%. Optimal oxygen therapy provides an adequate supply to ensure aerobic cellular metabolism or an arterial oxygen saturation (SaO2) above 85%.

   - Because the rate and depth of respirations for persons with chronic pulmonary obstructive disease (COPD) are governed by a degree of hypoxemia, only low dose oxygen is used (1-3 Liters/minute). Higher levels of oxygen delivery may decrease respiratory activity and possibly lead to respiratory failure and arrest.

— Pulse oximetry is a non-invasive technique for continuous monitoring of peripheral capillary saturation. A beam of light from a clip placed on an earlobe, finger or toe detects oxygen saturation that is translated into a digital reading on a bedside display.

— Transtracheal oxygen delivery is used for persons requiring long-term management. Lower doses can be administered during both phases of the ventilatory cycle. This method does not interfere with talking or drinking.

4. Chest tubes and suction

— Thoracotomy or chest tubes may be placed in the pleural space to remove air or fluid by a sterile, closed system (underwater seal) and sometimes indirect suction. Restoring negative pressure within the pleural space allows the lung to re-expand.

• Air accumulation is removed from the anterior (upper) tube and fluid from the posterior (lower) tube. The system includes 1-3 bottle set up or combined single units which are commercially available.

• The fluid level should rise in the tube with inspiration and fall during expiration. This fluctuation occurs until the lung is re-expanded.

— If a tube becomes disconnected or the collecting equipment is accidently broken, restoring a closed system as soon as possible is essential. There is controversy about the use of forceps to clamp the tubing. Some references say that clamping the tube near the chest prevents atmospheric air from entering the pleural space with respiratory activity. Other references say the clamping can increase air accumulation within the pleural space if a pleural tear or tension pneumothorax is present. A Heimlich valve is preferable to clamping.

— Clinical research studies have demonstrated that "stripping" or "milking" the tubes can cause varying amounts of negative pressure within the pleural space and may damage fragile pleural tissue. Thus, this intervention is no longer routinely done.

— Deep inspiration is very painful following chest surgery and chest tube placement. Shallow respiratory effort is common. Maintaining adequate pain control during the first 2-3 days post-op allows cooperation during coughing, breathing and mobilization activities. External splinting or support of the incision facilitates deeper inspiratory ability.

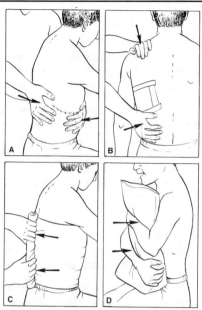

Fig. 2-9. **Splinting techniques.** *Apply firm, even pressure after the person has taken a deep breath and during forced expiratory cough. Do not squeeze the chest or interfere with chest inspiratory expansion. (A) Place one hand around the person's back and the other around the incisional area. (B) Support the area below the incision with one hand while exerting downward pressure on the shoulder on the affected side with the other. (C) Place a towel or draw sheet snugly (but not tightly) around the chest. (D) Have the person hug the pillow during forced expiratory cough. From J. Luckmann, K.C. Sorensen: Chapter 34-Nursing people experiencing chest surgery, <u>Medical-Surgical Nursing: A Psychophysiologic Approach</u>, 4th ed. (D. Kay, Ed.); Philadelphia: W.B. Saunders Company, 1993. Reprinted with permission.*

— Cessation of fluid fluctuation in the tubing and return of breath sounds over the involved area suggest re-expansion. Chest x-ray verifies re-expansion before tube removal.

  • Prior to the removal, the person should receive an adequate dose of analgesic 30 minutes before the physician removes the tube. After the suture securing the tube is cut, the person is asked to inhale deeply. The tube is then promptly removed. The site is covered with a Telfa dressing to ensure an airtight covering.

— Subcutaneous emphysema may occur near the tube insertion site, near a thoracic incision or following penetrating chest trauma. Small air bubbles are trapped in the subcutaneous tissue and palpated as a crackling sensation. The cause of the air leak must be identified and controlled. The trapped air is gradually absorbed and rarely causes physiological problems.

6. Medications

    — Antibiotic therapy is specific to the causative organism. Therefore, obtaining a sputum specimen prior to the initiation of broad spectrum antibiotic therapy is essential.

    — Bronchodilators are administered by several routes to relax bronchial smooth muscles, minimize airway spasms and relieve obstruction. As this category of medications has multiple physiological responses, side effects are common. Due to the concurrent stimulation of the central nervous system and cardiac activity, monitoring vital signs during repeated doses and intravenous administration is essential for early recognition of potentially severe side effects.

        • Aminophylline and theophylline are commonly prescribed for bronchodilating actions. These preparations can also markedly increase the heart rate and produce dysrhythmias.

        • Epinephrine may be administered to reverse severe bronchospasm and in an anaphylactic response.

        • Bronchodiltors (Ventolin, Alupent, Serevent, Bronkosol, Brethine) are commonly administered by metered-dose inhalation. Low dose steroids (Aerobid, Becolvent) may be administered concurrently. There are few systemic side effects from inhalation steroid therapy.

    — Mucokinetic agents alter the consistency of bronchial tree secretions and thereby facilitate their clearance with coughing or suctioning. Water and saline are used as diluents. Muco-lytics are substances which change the consistency of the secretions; e.g. N-acetylcysteine (Mucomyst).

SECTION 3: EXAMPLES OF COMMON ACUTE CLINICAL CONDITIONS

Acute Respiratory Failure

As pathophysiology of a pre-existing respiratory condition may become more involved, respiratory insufficiency may progress to respiratory failure and possibly arrest. Therefore, the astute medical-surgical nurse needs to establish a baseline of respiratory assessment data so that deviations can be identified and interventions to improve respiratory efficiency can be initiated early.

Two terms refer to ventilatory activity that does not permit adequate gas exchange in spite of spontaneous respiratory effort. These clinical situations are not interchangeable or equivalent to respiratory arrest (cessation of respiratory activity).

1. Respiratory insufficiency refers to an inadequate or borderline exchange of oxygen and/or carbon dioxide. With supplemental oxygen administration, minimal physical activities can be under-taken. Any additional activity or impairment of respiratory activity may precipitate respiratory failure.

2. Respiratory failure refers to exchange of oxygen and/or carbon dioxide outside acceptable levels. As references vary, the typical criteria for respiratory failure include the following arterial blood gas parameters: paO_2 below 50-60 mmHg; $paCO_2$ above 50 mmHg and SaO_2 below 80-85%. Mechanical ventilation is usually needed to correct this respiratory state and restore optimal gas exchange. If untreated, respiratory arrest (apnea) may result.

Acute Asthmatic Attack

This condition involves an acute, reversible narrowing of the upper airways (trachea and bronchi) and difficulty in breathing which is precipitated by a variety of factors. In addition to airway narrowing, the mucosa becomes edematous with increased mucus production. When an attack does not respond to treatment, a life-threatening prolonged attack may occur (status asthmaticus).

1. Attacks often occur at night with the person waking with a choking sensation. Initially the narrowing produces audible wheezing on expiration. As ventilatory effort becomes impaired, the rate and effort are noticeably increased and wheezing becomes audible on both inspiration and expiration.

   — Mouth breathing and nasal flaring become apparent. The person appears apprehensive, diaphoretic and focused on their breathing effort.

2. Bronchodilator medications administered by metered-dose inhaler early in an attack usually reverse symptoms. Oxygen by cannula minimizes secondary hypoxemia.

   — Moderate to severe attacks may require more aggressive therapy. If intravenous aminophylline is administered, cardiac monitoring is warranted as the tachycardia and dysrrhythmias are common. As the central nervous system is also stimulated with aminophylline, mild sedation may also be indicated.

     • Baseline serum theophylline levels are obtained before increasing dosage or changing preparations. Near toxic levels may occur in spite of appropriate self administration or without symptom relief. Therapeutic range is 10-20 ug/ml.

3. Cromolyn sodium and Nedocromil are benefical to prevent asthmatic attack and are administered by inhalation four times/day.

Lung Cancer (Bronchogenic Carcinoma)

For nearly 40 years, this form of cancer has been the leading cause of death among men. Since 1986, the incidence has progressively increased among women. Eighty to ninety percent of lung cancer occurs in persons who smoke tobacco, particularly cigarette smoking. Environmental and occupational exposure to chemical, toxins and pollutants also contribute to the incidence.

1. Most persons are asymptomatic in the early stages. Early indicators are often confused with other pulmonary conditions: persistent cough, sputum production, frequent respiratory infections. Associated weight loss indicates more advanced disease.

   — A change in the character of a chronic cough warrants further assessment.

2. Surgical removal of the tumor followed by chemotherapy is the usual treatment.

   — Pneumonectomy is the removal of one lung. Immediate postoperative nursing care includes the following:

     • Chest tubes are usually not placed on the operative side as there is no lung left to re-expand. Serous drainage will collect in the operated space. Gradually it will solidify and stabilize the chest wall.

     • The person is encouraged to lie on the back or operated side of facilitate maximum lung expansion and gas exchange on the unoperated lung. It usually takes 2-4 days following surgery for the remaining lung to accommodate the increase in blood flow; therefore there is a potential for fluid overload especially with intravenous therapy.

   — Lobectomy is the removal of one lobe of one lung; whereas segmental resection is the removal of a well-defined section of lung tissue. Immediate post-operative nursing care includes the following:

     • Chest tubes are placed in the pleural space to facilitate drainage and re-expansion of the remaining lung tissue. Monitoring vital signs in association with the amount of drainage from chest tubes provides assessment circulatory status and the early detection of post-operative hemorrhage.

- Chest surgery and placement of chest tubes are painful. Undermedication can impair sufficient depth of breathing and coughing activities and delay re-expansion. To facilitate effective cough, the incision should be supported anteriorly and posteriorly by the nurse or respiratory therapist.

Cancer of the Larynx

Squamous cell carcinoma of the larynx is increasing in the United States. It occurs most often in men over 60 years of age who have a history of heavy smoking, chronic laryngitis and vocal abuse.

1. Any smoker who becomes progressively hoarse or is hoarse longer than 2 weeks is urged to seek medical evaluation. If the tumor is limited to the true vocal chord, there is a 80-90% cure rate with surgical removal.

   - Hemilaryngectomy refers to the partial removal of the larynx or portion of a vocal cord. Minimal changes in swallowing and speaking are encountered post-operatively.

   - Total laryngectomy refers to complete excision of the larynx in which no connection between the trachea and the mouth exists post-operatively. A permanent tracheostomy is in place and the person has no natural voice.

   - Radical neck dissection may be performed along with a laryngectomy for persons with a high risk for metastases to the neck. In addition to a permanent tracheostomy, cervical lymph nodes, submandibular salivary glands and portions of the sternocleidomastoid muscle are removed. There is some visible alteration in physical appearance after healing.

2. Speech rehabilitation is possible for some persons by expelling swallowed air (esophageal speech). A hand-held, battery-operated artificial device assists others to produce a voice replication for audible communication.

3. With a permanent opening to the trachea, care must be taken to protect the lungs from aspiration of foreign materials and water when bathing or showering.

Pneumonia

This is an acute infection of lung tissue. It usually is caused by the inhalation of a specific bacteria, fungi or virus. Usually the disease process can be controlled by appropriate antibiotic therapy.

1. At risk clinical situations

    — Persons who are chronically ill or have lowered resistance are
    at risk for a minor upper respiratory tract infection which may
    progress to pneumonia (COPD, elderly). H. influenza and
    staphylococcus aureus organisms are particularly problematic
    for these persons.

    — Persons with altered immune states or receiving chemo-ther-
    apy are likely to develop opportunistic pneumonias. Pneu-
    mocystis carinii pneumonia is particularly problematic for
    persons with HIV or AIDS .

    — Persons with endotracheal or tracheostomy tubes are at risk
    for nosocomial infections from introduction of organisms into
    their artificial airway.

    — Persons who aspirate gastric contents into their trachea also
    inhale a variety of pathogens (*Klebsiella, Pseudomonas,
    Serratia, Escherichia* and *Proteus*) which require aggressive
    antibiotic therapy to control disease progression.

2. Clinical signs of developing pneumonia include: productive cough,
    change in the character or color of sputum production, elevating
    fever sometimes with chills, increase in auscultated lung sounds
    (congestion).

    — Pathogens may enter the pulmonary circulation and the infec-
    tion may develop into generalized sepsis.

Pulmonary Embolus

A pulmonary embolus occurs when a portion of a blood clot breaks
away and travels through the venous system and lodges in a pulmonary artery causing an occlusion. Blood flow is obstructed through
this vessel causing tissue hypoxia distal or beyond the point of obstruction. Other pulmonary vessels vasoconstrict which furthers the
pulmonary tissue hypoxemia.

1. Ventilation (breathing) is greater than the perfusion of blood within
    the pulmonary circulation (ventilation-perfusion mismatch).

    — If a large pulmonary artery is involved, the person will experi-
    ence sudden, sharp chest pain with severe dyspnea, coughing
    and hemoptysis. Shock may develop rapidly.

    — If a smaller artery is involved, symptoms will be less severe.
    The person will experience tachypnea (increased respirations),
    chest pain when inhaling, productive cough and a temperature
    elevation within 24 hours of the event. Adventitious breath
    sounds are heard on chest auscultation.

2. Anticoagulant therapy is prescribed to minimize the extension of the existing clot and minimize further fragmentation from the original clot. Heparin may be administered by continuous intravenous infusion with the dosage or flow rate regulated (titrated) according to scheduled partial thromboplastin times (PTT).

   — The goal of anticoagulant therapy is to prolong the time for clot formation. The desired PTT time in this clinical situation is 1.5-2 times normal values. Place this information in a clini-cal context. If the normal PTT values for an institution are 68-82 seconds, then 1.5-2 times normal or 100-180 seconds would be the criteria for titrating or adjusting the anticoagulant dosage to minimize the extension of a pulmonary embolus.

   — Thrombolytic therapy may be utilized to dissolve a massive embolus (urokinase, streptokinase).

   — Long-term maintenance anticoagulant therapy is achieved with oral preparations (Warfarin, Coumadin). Response to therapy is monitored by prothrombin times (PT).

3. Persons who are at risk for recurrence may have a filter placed inside their vena cava to catch fragments before they enter the right side of the heart and travel to the lungs.

Pneumothorax or Hemothorax

This is a condition in which air or blood collects in the pleural space to the extent that adjacent lung tissue is compressed and eventually collapses. Chest trauma and fractured ribs are the most common cause of pleural injury and lung collapse. However, weakened tissue from emphysema or acute asthma are predisposing factors.

Pneumothorax refers to air collection, whereas hemothorax refers to blood collection. Atelectasis refers to areas of collapsed lung tissue with or without associated pleural dysfunction.

1. Types

   — A spontaneous (closed) pneumothorax refers to sudden tear of the pleura or rupture of an air-filled blister (emphysematous bleb) on the surface on the lung. Air escapes from the lung tissue into the pleural space.

   — Tension pneumothorax refers to a one way air leak into the pleural space which increases in size with each breath. The chest tubes should not be clamped in this situation as lung collapse will rapidly reoccur.

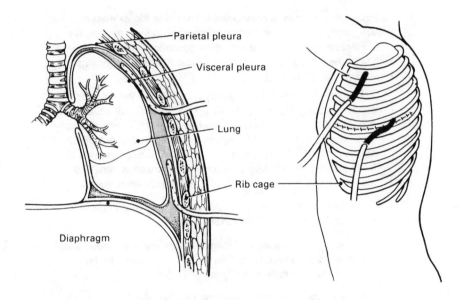

Fig. 2-10. Placement of chest tubes. From S.M. Lewis, I.C. Collier: Medical-Surgical Nursing: Assessment and Management of Clinical Problems, 4th ed.; St. Louis: Mosby-Year Book, Inc., 1995. Reprinted with permission.

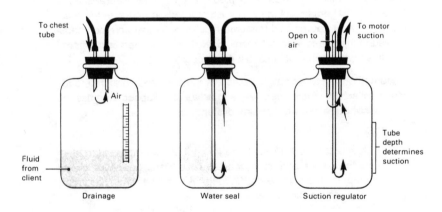

Fig. 2-11. Three-bottle water-seal suction. From S.M. Lewis, I.C. Collier: Medical-Surgical Nursing: Assessment and Management of Clinical Problems, 4th ed.; St. Louis: Mosby-Year Book, Inc., 1995. Reprinted with permission.

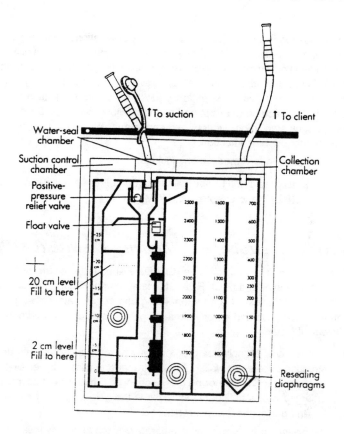

Fig. 2-12. Pleur-evac disposable chest suction system. From S.M. Lewis, I.C. Collier: Medical-Surgical Nursing: Assessment and Management of Clinical Problems, 4th ed.; St. Louis: Mosby-Year Book, Inc., 1995. Reprinted with permission.

2. Chest (thoracotomy) tubes are inserted to facilitate the removal of accumulated air or blood. The return of breath sounds over the involved area and the cessation of drainage or fluctuation are assessment data associated with lung re-expansion. X-ray will verify adequate re-expansion before the tubes are removed.

Tuberculosis (TB)

Although TB is considered a preventable and curable disease, it still requires public health attention. The organism can affect any body system but most commonly affects the lung tissue (pulmonary TB). The causative organism is a bacterium, mycobacterium tuberculosis, which usually responds favorably to specific medications.

The incidence is increasing among minority populations living in poverty living conditions. A drug resistant strain of mycobacterium is being identified among HIV positive persons who also have tuberculosis. It is speculated that drug resistant strains developed among noncompliant persons who intermittently took prescribed medications allowing the bacteria to adapt and change cellular structure. Drug resistant strains are more virulent and cause a rapidly developing and often life-threatening infection.

— The standard medications include:

isoniazid (INH); rifampin; ethambutol (EMB); pyrazinamide (PZA); and streptomycin (SM).

Chronic Obstructive Pulmonary Disease (COPD)

Chronic obstructive lung disease (COLD) is another term currently used for this syndrome. COPD/COLD is a primary cause of disability in the United States. It is an interrelating and degenerative triad of asthma, bronchitis and emphysema. Cigarette smoking is a primary etiological factor.

1. The terminal bronchioles progressively become enlarged with destruction of alveolar walls. Air is entrapped in dilated lower airways resulting in little or no gas exchange. The thorax becomes enlarged with a noticeable increase in the anterior-posterior diameter and barrel chest appearance.

   — Breathing becomes more labored with progressively less physical activity. Abdominal diaphragmatic breathing with forceful and prolonged exhalation increases the expiration of carbon dioxide retained in the lower airway. Pursed-lip breathing facilitates positive airways pressures and minimizes the collapse of the smaller ducts between each breath.

   — Due to the trapped air in the terminal airways, exhalation becomes progressively ineffective leading to the build up (accumulation) of carbon dioxide in the venous circulation. The kidneys compensate for the elevating respiratory acidosis by retaining bicarbonate (HCO^-) ions. A balanced or compensated acid-base state occurs.

   — With the persistent accumulation of carbon dioxide within the venous circulation, the primary stimulation of respiratory activity becomes diminished. The secondary stimulus, de-creased circulating oxygen levels, is activated for these individuals. This is an essential fact to remember when administering oxygen.

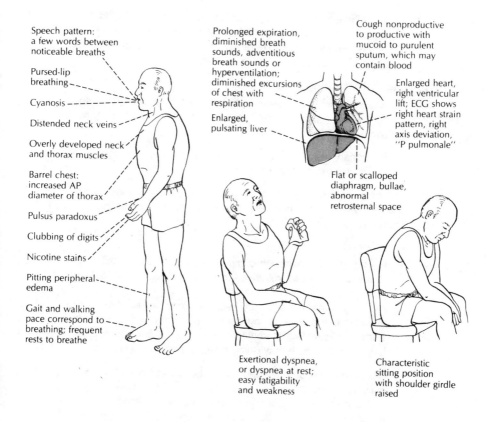

Speech pattern: a few words between noticeable breaths

Pursed-lip breathing

Cyanosis

Distended neck veins

Overly developed neck and thorax muscles

Barrel chest: increased AP diameter of thorax

Pulsus paradoxus

Clubbing of digits

Nicotine stains

Pitting peripheral edema

Gait and walking pace correspond to breathing; frequent rests to breathe

Prolonged expiration, diminished breath sounds, adventitious breath sounds or hyperventilation; diminished excursions of chest with respiration

Enlarged, pulsating liver

Cough nonproductive to productive with mucoid to purulent sputum, which may contain blood

Enlarged heart, right ventricular lift; ECG shows right heart strain pattern, right axis deviation, "P pulmonale"

Flat or scalloped diaphragm, bullae, abnormal retrosternal space

Exertional dyspnea, or dyspnea at rest; easy fatigability and weakness

Characteristic sitting position with shoulder girdle raised

Fig. 2-13. COPD/COLD changes. From J. Luckmann, K.C. Sorensen: Chapter 32- Nursing people experiencing lower airway disorders, Medical-Surgical Nursing: A Psycho-physiologic Approach, 4th ed. (D. Kay, Ed.); Philadelphia: W.B. Saunders Company, 1993. Reprinted with permission.

— With the persistent accumulation of carbon dioxide within the venous circulation, the primary stimulation of respiratory activity becomes diminished. The secondary stimulus, decreased circulating oxygen levels, is activated for these individuals. This is an essential fact to remember when administering oxygen.

• Low doses (1-3 Liters/minute) of oxygen may be needed during minimal physical activity, but higher doses (over 5 Liters/minute) may diminish their stimulus for respiratory activity.

- Air pollutants may trigger an asthmatic attack, causing acute bronchospasm and increase bronchial secretions. Narrowed airways and increased secretions further impair exhalation of carbon dioxide and inhalation of oxygen.

2. Diagnostic findings
   - Arterial blood gas analysis indicates chronic respiratory acidosis ($paCO_2$ greater than 45 mmHg) with metabolic compensation (HCO_3 greater than 26 mEq/Liter).

   - Pulmonary function studies indicate increased respiratory effort with increased residual volume.

3. The goals of management of care focus on (1) improving gas exchange, (2) removing bronchial secretions and (3) preventing brochopulmonary infections.

4. Complications
   - Pneumonia is a common complication due to decreased respiratory effectiveness, retained bronchial secretions and lowered resistance to infections. Individuals with COPD learn to detect the early signs of respiratory tract infections by identifying changes in the color, amount and consistency of their sputum. Early administration of antibiotics can divert a serious respiratory infection which may quickly lead to respiratory failure.

   - Cor pulmonale is right sided congestive heart failure that results from chronic respiratory dysfunction. The physiological response to prolonged serum elevation of carbon dioxide is vasoconstriction of the pulmonary arteries. The subsequent pulmonary vascular hypertension increases the workload of the right side of the heart. As the workload increases there is progressive congestion in the venous system. (Refer to Unit 3 for additional discussion of right-sided congestive heart failure.)

   - Hepatomegaly or enlarged liver may occur when persistent venous congestion backs up from the right side of the heart. Due to elevated vascular pressure within the liver, fluid may shift into the peritoneal cavity (ascites). The combination of an enlarged liver and ascites often elevates the diaphragm and further compromises respiratory effectiveness.

Focused Bedside Assessment

The following data would be expected from a head-to-toe assessment of an individual admitted with an acute episode of COPD. No other patho-physiological problems involving other body system dysfunction unrelated to COPD is included.

* **General appearance:** Weak, fatigued, skeletal muscle wasting, varying degrees of respiratory distress.

* **Neurological status:** Fluctuates between alert/oriented to lethargy/confusion. When respiratory acidosis is present, lethargy and drowsiness are commonly observed. When hypoxemia is present, restlessness, irritability and confusion are commonly observed.

* **Cardiac status:** The ability of the heart to pump blood from the right side of the heart through the lungs and out into general circulation becomes impaired (cor pulmonale).

  Cardiac rate generally increases in response to hypoxemia. Chest pain and dysrrhythmias may occur subsequent to decreased myocardial perfusion and decreased oxygenated blood supply.

* **Respiratory status:** Varying degrees of dyspnea occur in response to physical activity. Progressive respiratory effort with increased use of accessory muscles such as mouth breathing and clavicular rise occur.

  Abdominal breathing becomes automatic. Forceful coughing episodes especially after being supine are common. Yellow, green or blood tinged sputum warrants analysis for the causative organism.

  Lung sounds are distant with varying degrees of congestion.

* **Abdominal status:** Soft and distended when ascites is present. Bowel sounds present but diminished. An enlarged liver may be palpated below the right lower rib margin. Further assessment of possible liver dysfunction is warranted when heptomegaly is identified.

* **Urinary status:** Urinary elimination patterns normally are unchanged. However, as COPD is common among middle to older men who may also have benign prostatic hypertrophy, urinary tract infections may develop. Refer to Unit 6 for additional information of prostatic conditions.

* **Extremities:** If general perfusion is diminished, peripheral pulses remain present but feet and hands may be cool to touch.

  When cor pulmonale is present, impaired venous return may lead to dependent edema in lower extremities or at the sacrum in bedfast persons.

* When the individual is turned on their side, the nurse would expect to find: congestion in both lung fields consistent with the anterior findings. If the individual has been in bed, dependent edema may be noted in the sacral area.

If additional data are observed, a more detailed assessment of the involved system is required. Additional areas of physiological dysfunction may be present and confound the present respiratory problem.

Ventilatory Dependent

Some persons are unable to sustain adequate gas exchange in spite of spontaneous respiratory effort. Their respiratory status is inadequate but stable and often cared for on an intermediate medical-surgical nursing unit, in long-term facilities or at home. Persons who are ventilatory dependent may be alert and oriented or comatose. In spite of their respiratory inadequacy, the physiological functioning of other body systems may be within normal limits (WNL).

1. Mechanical ventilation may be administered continuously or with scheduled "on-off" routines.

2. Chronic respiratory inefficiency and inadequacy may be due to:
   - Depressed central nervous system function (coma) resulting in shallow breathing and ineffective cough response.

   - Paralysis of intercostal muscles resulting in only diaphragmatic activity and ineffective cough response (high spinal cord injuries).

   - Severely weakened skeletal muscles resulting in shallow respirations and ineffective cough response (neurogenic respiratory conditions).

   - Severely damaged lung tissue resulting in ineffective exhalation of carbon dioxide (COPD/COLD).

   - Morbid obesity (Pickwickian syndrome) in which the individual's tidal volume is no longer adequate for their body size.

3. Efforts to wean these individuals from mechanical ventilation may be unsuccessful to date. Weaning efforts will continue but long term mechanical ventilation via a tracheostomy is warranted.
   - These individuals may have adequate cognitive abilities, be awake, alert and oriented. They just are unable to adequately breath or exchange oxygen and/or carbon dioxide.

   - They are at risk for secondary respiratory infections (pneumonia) and immobility complications.

4. Drug resistant infections are increasing and becoming life threatening. Methicillin resistant staphylococcus aureaus (MRSA) is seen as active disease process in acute care, home health and nursing home settings especially among ventilatory dependent persons. Vancomycin is the antibiotic of choice for drug resistant infections. However, organisms are becoming resistant to this drug and other serious infections result. VRE refers to vancomycin resistant enterococci infection and no antibiotic is currently effective in treating this life threatening infection.

5. The presence of drug resistant organisms have been found in individuals who do not have clinical symptoms. Colonization refers to the process by which these organisms are present in a symptom free individual but can be passed on to a susceptible individual. Colonization presents a significant health problem in the control of drug resistant infections.

unit *3*

NURSING CARE OF ADULTS WITH

Circulatory Conditions

T *his unit addresses common and stable circulatory conditions of adults which involve the heart, blood vessels and blood components that are cared for on general medical-surgical nursing units. The management and care of critical and unstable conditions, such as acute myocardial infarction, cardiogenic shock or immediate post-operative care for by-pass surgery or valve replacement, are not included. The interpretation and management of cardiac dysrhythmias also are not addressed as these situations require continuous cardiac monitoring.*

Persons with an acute unstable circulatory problem are usually admitted to specialty-care units where cardiac and hemodynamic functions are closely monitored. However, some persons on a general medical-surgical nursing unit are at risk for an acute circulatory episode. It is important for the nurses on these units to recognize situations which may alter circulatory homeostasis. The recognition of the signs and symptoms of changes in perfusion and early initiation of interventions minimize the development of a circulatory crisis.

SECTION 1: OVERVIEW

The nursing care of adults with circulatory dysfunction encompasses a wide variety of pathophysiological conditions. Effective plans for care are based upon an understanding of the normal functions of the heart, blood vessels and blood components.

Anatomical Considerations

1. The cardiovascular system consists of an efficient pump (heart), an elaborate interconnecting system of tubing (vessels) and efficient carriers of the nutrients for cellular metabolism (blood components).

2. Heart

    — The heart is divided into four chambers: two atria and two ventricles. The chambers are separated by valves which keep the blood in the appropriate compartments. They open and close at appropriate times during the cardiac cycle, permitting the forward flow of blood.

    — The heart is functionally divided into two sides: a right side and a left side. The right heart receives blood from the venous system and circulates it to the lungs. The left heart receives oxygenated blood from the lungs and pumps it out into the systemic circulation.

3. Blood vessels

    — As a general rule, arteries carry oxygenated blood and nutrients from the heart, and veins carry the waste products of cellular metabolism from the tissue and back to the heart. There are only two exceptions. The pulmonary artery carries deoxygenated blood from the right ventricle to the lungs, and the pulmonary vein carries oxygenated blood from the lungs to the left atrium of the heart.

    — The arteries which supply the heart muscle (myocardium) branch off the aorta immediately outside of the left ventricle. The coronary arteries lie on the surface of the heart and fill during the resting phase of the cardiac cycle (diastole).

    — A network of tiny blood vessels (capillaries) connect the arteries and veins and comprise the microcirculation. The walls of these vessels are a single layer of cells which allow for the exchange of gases and small nutrient molecules.

    — There are more veins than arteries; therefore, the venous system contains more circulating blood. Movement through the veins back toward the heart is dependent upon extravascular pressures from body tissues, muscles and intravascular valves.

4. Blood components

    — Blood is an aqueous solution (plasma) that contains proteins, electrolytes, inorganic and organic constituents. The solids which make up only a small portion of the blood, are measured by a percentage value or hematocrit (Hct).

    — The cellular components of the blood include erythrocytes (red blood cells), leukocytes (white blood cells) and thrombocytes (platelets). These cells are produced in the bone marrow of the skull, vertebrae, pelvis, sternum, ribs and the end of long bones. Production (hematopoiesis) occurs in a regular cycle or in response to blood loss or cell destruction.

    — Red blood cells (RBC) are soft, pliable disk-shaped cells. New, immature red blood cells in circulation are called reticulocytes, and normally there are only a few in the circulation.

    — There are several types of white blood cells (WBCs), each having a distinct function. New, immature WBCs in circulation are called bands, and normally there are only a few in circulation.

Normal Physiological Functioning

1. General considerations

    — The cardiovascular and pulmonary systems are closely interrelated for the purpose of gas exchange between the lungs and tissues. This unity is referred to as cardiopulmonary function.

    — There is also a unity of function between the cardiovascular system and the blood components for the delivery or perfusion of nutrients and essential elements to body organs and tissue for optimal cellular metabolism.

2. Cardiac physiology (cardiac cycle)

    — Cardiac function involves interrelationships among; (1) electrical impulse transmission, (2) valve effectiveness, (3) pump efficiency, and (4) circulation to the heart muscle. Any dysfunction of one component will affect the function of another component.

    — The pumping capacity of the heart is governed by the electrical impulses and the contraction of cardiac muscle. Adequate amounts of potassium, calcium and magnesium are needed for normal sequence of transmission and contraction.

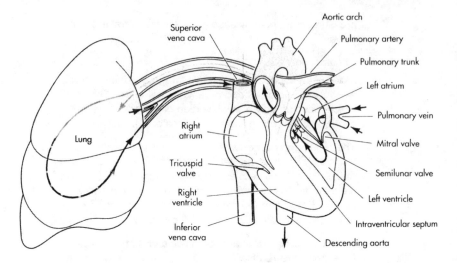

Fig. 3-1. Schematic representation of blood flow through the heart. Arrows indicate direction of flow. S.M. Lewis, I.C. Collier: Medical-Surgical Nursing: Assessment and Management of Clinical Problems, 4th ed.; St. Louis: Mosby-Year Book, Inc., 1995. Reprinted with permission.

- The cardiac impulse begins in the sino-atrial (SA) node in the right atrium of the heart. The impulse travels to the atrio-ventricular (AV) node and then along the neural fibers in the ventricular muscle wall of the heart. The visualization of electrical impulse transmission is recorded as an electrocardiogram (ECG or EKG).

- Atria contract in response to the atrial segment of impulse transmission and blood flows into the ventricles. In a similar manner, ventricles contract in response to the ventricular segment of impulse transmission. Blood leaves the heart from the ventricles and flows to the lungs and the periphery.

- Valves are located throughout the cardiovascular system to ensure the forward flow of blood. Valves located in the heart and major vessels keep blood in the appropriate compartments. The closing of valves in the heart are heard as a heart beat.

- The heart is a fascinating muscular structure which quickly responds to organ and tissue needs by changing the rate or force of contractions. The heart pumps one burst of blood with each heartbeat. The volume pumped per minute or cardiac output (CO) can be calculated and adjusted according to body weight (cardiac index or CI).

Flow of cardiac impulse

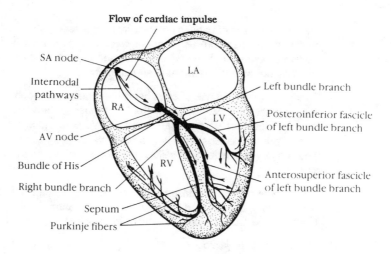

Fig. 3-2. Conduction system of the heart. Modified from M. Kinney and others: Comprehensive Cardiac Care, 8th ed.; St. Louis: Mosby-Year Book, Inc., 1996. Reprinted with permission.

3. Vascular physiology
   - Arteries are elastic vessels which stretch to accommodate the volume of blood which passes through them en route toward the tissues. Their ability to constrict offers varying degrees of resistance against which the heart must pump. This mechanism is called systemic vascular resistance (SVR).

   - The ability of arteries to change their diameter is a response to various physiological processes to redirect blood flow according to metabolic need. For example, constricting the blood flow to the extremities in a state of shock allows the arteries in the heart muscle, brain and kidneys to dilate and receive an adequate blood supply.

   - The wave of blood flow through the arteries is recorded as blood pressure. The peak or highest reading is the systolic blood pressure. The lowest point, diastolic blood pressure, occurs between waves and when the heart is at rest. The difference between the highest (systole) and the lowest (diastole) reading is the pulse pressure.

   - The wave of pressure through the peripheral arteries is palpated or felt as a pulse. Normally, the heart rate and the pulse rate are the same numerical value.

- The effectiveness of cardiac contractility is assessed by the quality of peripheral pulses. A strong force of ventricular contraction produces a strong peripheral pulse. A weak contraction may not be felt (palpated) in an extremity.

- During the resting phase of each heart beat (diastole), blood flows into the arteries that supply the heart muscle. Because the heart does not store oxygen or nutrients, a constant supply is required. Any alteration in the coronary vasculature affects the coronary circulation and cellular metabolism of the heart muscle.

- The amount of oxygen consumed or utilized by the heart is dependent upon the rate and force of myocardial contractions. The term, cardiac workload, is used in this context.

4. Blood component physiology

- Hemoglobin (Hgb), a major component of the RBC, transports oxygen and carbon dioxide between the lungs and the tissues.

- Several elements are required for normal RBC production (erythropoiesis) including Vitamin B_{12}, folic acid, iron, copper, and the hormone erythropoietin. RBCs circulate for 120 days and are then dismantled. Some elements are excreted and others are recycled into new RBCs.

- White blood cells (WBC or leukocytes) include a variety of cells which participate in the inflammatory and immune responses. WBCs include monocytes, lymphocytes, neutrophils, basophils and esinophils. The most important WBC function is to defend the body against foreign invasion by producing and transporting defensive elements.

- Platelets are cell fragments which are essential for blood clot formation (coagulation). Platelets collect and attach to damaged vessels to control bleeding. They are also essential in the cascade of factors involved in the coagulation mechanism.

Variations Related to Aging

Much controversy exists regarding the effects of normal aging on the cardiovascular system. Thus, separating the physiological changes of aging from the changes due to the presence of atherosclerosis is difficult. The complications secondary to atherosclerosis are also prevalent among the elderly and account for the majority of deaths in this age group. Perhaps the modification of CV risk factors also apply to the elderly.

1. Despite changes due to aging, the heart can meet the day-to-day
    activities. It is only when increased physiological stress is present
    or prolonged that deteriorating function becomes apparent for the
    normal elderly person.

2. Thickening of the cardiac valves is common and may lead to sys-
    tolic murmurs. Asymptomatic valve disease from streptococcal in-
    fection during youth can be aggravated when increased cardiac
    workload is required during other body system dysfunction. Per-
    sons with this health history are at risk for left-sided congestive
    heart failure.

3. Concurrent presence of normal aging and atherosclerotic vessel dis-
    ease compromises coronary circulation. Acute angina or heart at-
    tack may occur during the management of other problems.
    Compromised coronary perfusion can impair pumping capacity
    and lead to chronic right-sided heart failure.

4. Management of hypertension is an ongoing goal. It is essential to
    determine each person's baseline blood pressure. A change of
    20 mm Hg for a hypertensive person may go undetected as an
    early sign of altered perfusion.

5. Blood composition changes little with age, although iron deficiency
    anemia is frequent. Erythrocyte life span remains unchanged but
    there is a delay in RBC production after blood loss which may be
    due to iron deficiency.

6. The number of lymphocytes does not change but their function
    decreases. There is a decreased ability to respond to antigens
    which may delay the onset of symptoms of infection as well as
    delay healing.

7. There is no decrease in the number of platelets but there is
    evidence of increased platelet adhesiveness which may lead to
    clot formation in various vessels.

SECTION 2: CARDIAC/CIRCULATORY DYSFUNCTION

Overview of Disrupted Function

In the United States, cardiovascular (CV) disease causes more deaths than all other diseases. The most common cause of death from heart disease after the age of 25 years is coronary atherosclerotic heart disease. More than one in four adults have some form of cardiovascular disease which also includes hypertensive heart disease, rheumatic heart disease and cerebrovascular disease. In the past decade, there has been a reduction in mortality which suggests that screening for early detection and public education of preventive measures are effective.

Risk Factors

1. Risk for the development of cardiac problems

    — Examine yourself and those persons to whom you are providing care. Identify their risk for developing cardiac/circulatory problems. According to the American Heart Association, a numerical score can be calculated which is predictive of an individual's risk for developing cardiac problems. Complete the assessment guide on the following pages.

2. Risk for the development of an acute cardiac/circulatory problem among non-cardiac persons

    — Persons with an acute unstable cardiac problem are usually admitted to specialty units where cardiac function is closely monitored. However, at-risk persons may be admitted to a general medical-surgical nursing unit for a non-cardiac/ circulatory problem, such as hernia repair or kidney stones. These individuals may also have asymptomatic circulatory-perfusion problems which are in physiological balance. Relatively minor deviations in health status may disrupt homeo-stasis and precipitate an acute circulatory episode. It is important for the non-critical care nurse to recognize at-risk persons and situations that may alter an individual's perfusion balance.

    Under most circumstances, these situations can be modified. The severity of cardiac dysfunction and the development of complications can be averted.

Fig. 3-3. **American Heart Association Risk Assessment**

MEN

Find the column for your age group. Everyone starts
with a score of 10 points. Work down the page *adding* points to your score or *subtracting* points from
your score.

		54 OR YOUNGER	55 OR OLDER

1. WEIGHT

Locate your weight category in the table below. If
you are in

		STARTING SCORE **10**	STARTING SCORE **10**
	weight category A	SUBTRACT 2	SUBTRACT 2
	weight category B	SUBTRACT 1	ADD 0
	weight category C	ADD 1	ADD 1
	weight category D	ADD 2	ADD 3

EQUALS ☐   EQUALS ☐

2. SYSTOLIC BLOOD PRESSURE

Use the "first" or "higher" number from your most
recent blood pressure measurement. If you do not
know your blood pressure, estimate it by using the
letter for your weight category. If your blood
pressure is

A	119 or less	SUBTRACT 1	SUBTRACT 5
	between 120 and 139	ADD 0	SUBTRACT 2
	between 140 and 159	ADD 0	ADD 1
	160 or greater	ADD 1	ADD 4

EQUALS ☐   EQUALS ☐

3. BLOOD CHOLESTEROL LEVEL

Use the number from your most recent blood
cholesterol test. If you do not know your blood
cholesterol, estimate it by using the letter for your
weight category. If your blood cholesterol is

A	199 or less	SUBTRACT 2	SUBTRACT 1
	between 200 and 224	SUBTRACT 1	SUBTRACT 1
	between 225 and 249	ADD 0	ADD 0
	250 or higher	ADD 1	ADD 0

EQUALS ☐   EQUALS ☐

4. CIGARETTE SMOKING

If you

(If you smoke a pipe, but not cigarettes, use the
same score adjustment as those cigarette smokers
who smoke less than a pack a day.)

	do not smoke	SUBTRACT 1	SUBTRACT 2
	smoke less than a pack a day	ADD 0	SUBTRACT 1
	smoke a pack a day	ADD 1	ADD 0
	smoke more than a pack a day	ADD 2	ADD 3

FINAL SCORE EQUALS ☐   FINAL SCORE EQUALS ☐

WEIGHT TABLE FOR MEN	YOUR HEIGHT FT IN	WEIGHT CATEGORY (lbs.)				
		A				
Look for your height (without shoes) in the far left column and then read across to find the category into which your weight (in indoor clothing) would fall.	5 1	up to 123	124-148	149-173	174 plus	
	5 2	up to 126	127-152	153-178	179 plus	Because both blood pressure and blood cholesterol are related to weight, an estimate of these risk factors for each weight category is printed at the bottom of the table.
	5 3	up to 129	130-156	157-182	183 plus	
	5 4	up to 132	133-160	161-186	187 plus	
	5 5	up to 135	136-163	164-190	191 plus	
	5 6	up to 139	140-168	169-196	197 plus	
	5 7	up to 144	145-174	175-203	204 plus	
	5 8	up to 148	149-179	180-209	210 plus	
	5 9	up to 152	153-184	185-214	215 plus	
	5 10	up to 157	158-190	191-221	222 plus	
	5 11	up to 161	162-194	195-227	228 plus	
	6 0	up to 165	166-199	200-232	233 plus	
	6 1	up to 170	171-205	206-239	240 plus	
	6 2	up to 175	176-211	212-246	247 plus	
	6 3	up to 180	181-217	218-253	254 plus	
	6 4	up to 185	186-223	224-260	261 plus	
	6 5	up to 190	191-229	230-267	268 plus	
	6 6	up to 195	196-235	236-274	275 plus	
ESTIMATE OF SYSTOLIC BLOOD PRESSURE		or less				
ESTIMATE OF BLOOD CHOLESTEROL		199 or less				

Courtesy American Heart Association.

WOMEN

Find the column for your age group. Everyone starts with a score of 10 points. Work down the page *adding* points to your score or *subtracting* points from your score.

	54 OR YOUNGER	55 OR OLDER

1. WEIGHT

Locate your weight category in the table below. If you are in . . .

	STARTING SCORE [10]	STARTING SCORE [10]
weight category A	SUBTRACT 2	SUBTRACT 2
weight category B	SUBTRACT 1	SUBTRACT 1
weight category C	ADD 1	ADD 1
weight category D	ADD 2	ADD 1
	EQUALS [ ]	EQUALS [ ]

2. SYSTOLIC BLOOD PRESSURE

Use the "first" or "higher" number from your most recent blood pressure measurement. If you do not know your blood pressure, estimate it by using the letter for your weight category. If your blood pressure is . . .

A	119 or less	SUBTRACT 2	SUBTRACT 3
	between 120 and 139	SUBTRACT 1	ADD 0
	between 140 and 159	ADD 0	ADD 3
	160 or greater	ADD 1	ADD 6
		EQUALS [ ]	EQUALS [ ]

3. BLOOD CHOLESTEROL LEVEL

Use the number from your most recent blood cholesterol test. If you do not know your blood cholesterol, estimate it by using the letter for your weight category. If your blood cholesterol is . . .

A	199 or less	SUBTRACT 1	SUBTRACT 3
	between 200 and 224	ADD 0	SUBTRACT 1
	between 225 and 249	ADD 0	ADD 1
	250 or higher	ADD 1	ADD 3
		EQUALS [ ]	EQUALS [ ]

4. CIGARETTE SMOKING

If you . . .

	do not smoke	SUBTRACT 1	SUBTRACT 2
	smoke less than a pack a day	ADD 0	SUBTRACT 1
	smoke a pack a day	ADD 1	ADD 1
	smoke more than a pack a day	ADD 2	ADD 4
		FINAL SCORE EQUALS [ ]	FINAL SCORE EQUALS [ ]

WEIGHT TABLE FOR WOMEN	YOUR HEIGHT FT IN	WEIGHT CATEGORY (lbs.)			
		A	B		
Look for your height (without shoes) in the far left column and then read across to find the category into which your weight (in indoor clothing) would fall.	4 8	up to 101	102-122	123-143	144 plus
	4 9	up to 103	104-125	126-146	147 plus
	4 10	up to 106	107-128	129-150	151 plus
	4 11	up to 109	110-132	133-154	155 plus
	5 0	up to 112	113-136	137-158	159 plus
	5 1	up to 115	116-139	140-162	163 plus
	5 2	up to 119	120-144	145-168	169 plus
	5 3	up to 122	123-148	149-172	173 plus
	5 4	up to 127	128-154	155-179	180 plus
	5 5	up to 131	132-158	*59-185	186 plus
	5 6	up to 135	136-163	164-190	191 plus
	5 7	up to 139	140-168	169-196	197 plus
	5 8	up to 143	144-173	174-202	203 plus
	5 9	up to 147	148-178	179-207	208 plus
	5 10	up to 151	152-182	183-213	214 plus
	5 11	up to 155	156-187	188-218	219 plus
	6 0	up to 159	160-191	192-224	225 plus
	6 1	up to 163	164-196	197-229	230 plus
ESTIMATE OF SYSTOLIC BLOOD PRESSURE		119 or less			
ESTIMATE OF BLOOD CHOLESTEROL		199 or less	200		

Because both blood pressure and blood cholesterol are related to weight, an estimate of these risk factors for each weight category is printed at the bottom of the table.

WHAT YOUR SCORE MEANS

0-4	You have one of the lowest risks of heart disease for your age and sex
5-9	You have a low to moderate risk of heart disease for your age and sex but there is some room for improvement
10-14	You have a moderate to high risk of heart disease for your age and sex, with considerable room for improvement on some factors
15-19	You have a high risk of developing heart disease for your age and sex with a great deal of room for improvement on all factors
20 & over	You have a very high risk of developing heart disease for your age and sex and should take immediate action on all risk factors

WARNING

* If you have diabetes, gout or a family history of heart disease, your actual risk will be greater than indicated by this appraisal.
* If you do not know your current blood pressure or blood cholesterol level you should visit your physician or health center to have them measured. Then figure your score again for a more accurate determination of your risk
* If you are overweight, have high blood pressure or high blood cholesterol, or smoke cigarettes, your long-term risk of heart disease is increased even if your risk in the next several years is low

HOW TO REDUCE YOUR RISK

* Try to quit smoking permanently. There are many programs available.
* Have your blood pressure checked regularly, preferably every twelve months after age 40. If your blood pressure is high, see your physician Remember blood pressure medicine is only effective if taken regularly
* Consider your daily exercise (or lack of it). A half hour of brisk walking, swimming or other enjoyable activity should not be difficult to fit into your day.
* Give some serious thought to your diet. If you are overweight, or eat a lot of foods high in saturated fat or cholesterol (whole milk, cheese, eggs, butter, fatty foods, fried foods) then changes should be made in your diet. Look for the *American Heart Association Cookbook* at your local bookstore

* Visit or write your local Heart Association for further information and copies of free pamphlets on many related subjects including
  * Reducing your risk of heart attack
  * Controlling high blood pressure
  * Eating to keep your heart healthy
  * How to stop smoking
  * Exercising for good health

SOME WORDS OF CAUTION

* If you have diabetes, gout, or a family history of heart disease, your real risk of developing heart disease will be greater than indicated by your RISKO score. If your score is high and you have one or more of these additional problems, you should give particular attention to reducing your risk

* If you are a woman under 45 years or a man under 35 years of age, your RISKO score represents an upper limit on your real risk of developing heart disease. In this case, your real risk is probably lower than indicated by your score.
* Using your weight category to estimate your systolic blood pressure or your blood cholesterol level makes your RISKO score less accurate.

* Your score will tend to overestimate your risk if your actual values on these two important factors are average for someone of your height and weight
* Your score will underestimate your risk if your actual blood pressure or cholesterol level is above average for someone of your height or weight

The following examples are common clinical situations that may disrupt homeostasis and may lead to an acute circulatory episode:

* Fluid imbalances; i.e. fluid overload or dehydration.

* Electrolyte imbalances; i.e. potassium, sodium, calcium, magnesium.

* High cellular metabolic needs; i.e. fever, draining wounds, burns.

* Poorly-controlled diabetes mellitus or hypertension.

The following examples are clinical situations that may precipitate cardiac dysrhythmias:

* Injured or damaged heart valves.

* Tissue hypoxia, particularly myocardial hypoxia. Chest pain may not always accompany cardiac hypoxia especially in the elderly, fainting may be the only symptom of a "silent MI."

* Sudden changes in blood pressure.

* Electrolyte imbalances, especially potassium, calcium and magnesium which are required for normal impulse transmission and muscle contraction.

Assessment of Circulatory/Perfusion Status

When the intravascular volume decreases or tissues require additional metabolic nutrients, the heart compensates by increasing its rate. The ability of the heart to sustain this compensating response is dependent upon the physical fitness of the heart and the presence of any cardiac pathology.

At some point, the heart can no longer meet the metabolic needs required by the cells. Then the heart begins to fail producing characteristic clinical manifestations of impaired perfusion and tissue hypoxia. Utilizing a systematic decision-making sequence is helpful to prioritize data and initiate independent and collaborative nursing action. By comparing observed data to an individual's baseline, trends and changes are recognized. Data also are the criteria for determining the effectiveness of specific interventions and plans for care.

Primary Sources of Data

1. Heart sounds

   — The closing of the valves of the heart is distinctly heard as "lub-dub" and described as S1 and S2 heart sounds. The contracting phase (systole) is a shorter phase than the resting phase (diastole). Therefore, the pause between S1 and S2 is shorter

than the pause between S2 and S1. Any additional sounds
or changes in this sequence are abnormal.

— A person may experience extra heart beats and describe them
as "palpitations," "skipping" or "thumping." This subjective
symptom may be detected by the bedside nurse as an irregularity in the peripheral pulse rhythm. An EKG confirms the
presence of an underlying dysrhythmia.

— A murmur is the auscultated sound of abnormal blood movement within the heart. For example, the back flow of blood
through insufficient heart valves produces a murmur. With clinical experience and the guidance of a mentor, the bedside
nurse gains clinical competence in recognizing the variations
in heart sounds.

2. Chest pain

— As you recall from the previous section in this unit, the heart
rests between ventricular contractions and blood flows into the
coronary arteries. When insufficient oxygen or nutrients are
delivered to the heart muscle, myocardial hypoxia develops.
Chest pain is the characteristic symptom of this pathophysiological state (myocardial tissue hypoxia).

— Clarification of the precipitating circumstances, onset and description of the pain, response to activity and interventions are
important in determining the cause of the chest pain.

— As pain is a subjective symptom, the intensity is best determined by the person experiencing it. The person is asked to
rate their pain from 1 to 10 with 10 being the most intense
pain ever experienced. Self-assessment coupled with clinical
manifestations of impaired perfusion provides a comprehensive perspective for the bedside nurse.

3. Level of Consciousness

— The brain requires approximately 15-20% of the blood
pumped from the heart with each beat. Therefore, when this
volume is not delivered to the brain, subtle changes in the
level of consciousness appear.

— Episodes of dizziness or fainting (syncope) especially when
bending over may be related to inadequate cardiac output or
narrowed carotid arteries (carotid insufficiency).

Fig. 3-4. Decision Tree for Acute Chest Pain

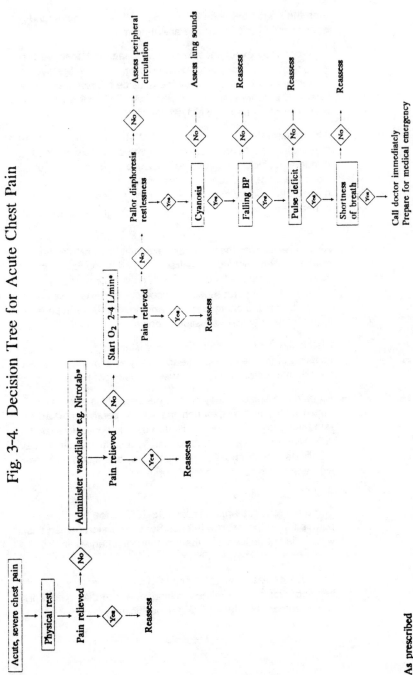

* As prescribed

- An acute inadequate supply of oxygenated blood to the brain produces restlessness, agitation or confusion. Whereas, a gradual decreasing blood supply produces drowsiness and lethargy. Sometimes a person may experience alternating periods of adequate and inadequate supply which produce a mixed pattern of clinical manifestations.

4. Cardiac output

   - As the strength of ventricular contractions diminishes, the volume of blood pumped from the heart diminishes. Without invasive hemodynamic monitoring, the bedside nurse must utilize other physiological clues to determine the extent of the perfusion deficit.

   - Fatigability is a subtle symptom to be monitored. Relatively minor increases in physical activity result in increased respiratory effort. Heart rate quickly increases with impaired peripheral perfusion.

   - In severe cases of decreased cardiac output, the person attempting minimal activity quickly becomes exhausted. The respiratory rate increases but is shallow and the heart rate increases but is weak. The person appears pale, diaphoretic with decreasing alertness. They appear to wilt like a fragile flower.

   - As cardiac output diminishes, perfusion to the kidney becomes impaired which triggers a powerful vasoconstricting response, the renin-angiotensin cycle. The arteries constrict and the systemic vascular resistance (SVR) increases and the heart must pump harder to move the blood into circulation.

   - If the heart is unable to work harder, a vicious cycle of decreased renal perfusion, vasoconstriction, tissue hypoxia and pain spirals. The physiological stress response accentuates this cycle.

5. Peripheral perfusion

   - Peripheral vasoconstriction is another physiological response to a decrease in cardiac output. This response is an attempt to maintain a blood pressure within normal limits (WNL).

   - Normally, arterial blood pressure accommodates for changes between lying, sitting and standing positions. Orthostatic (postural) hypotension refers to a sudden drop in blood pressure when a person rapidly moves from a sitting to a standing position.

   - Side effects of certain medications, especially anti-hypertensive agents may produce postural hypotension. Protection from injury due to fainting is a concern if this symptom is a possibility.

— As cardiac output decreases, the quality of peripheral pulses diminishes and is described as weak or thready. A wave of blood flow not detected by palpation produces an irregular pulse rhythm. In this situation, an apical heart rate should be assessed simultaneously with a peripheral pulse. A difference in rates suggests perfusion dysfunction or cardiac dysrhythmia.

— Difficulty locating a peripheral pulse may be due to diminished blood flow or edema over the pulse site. The use of a device (doppler) to magnify the sounds of blood movement may be helpful. Comparison of pulses in extremities may reveal a unilateral circulatory problem.

— Turbulent blood flow caused by a damaged valve or an abnormal opening between an artery and vein can be felt as a "thrill." Whereas, auscultation of turbulent blood flow is described as a "bruit."

6. Capillary refill
— Assessment of capillary refill is determined by pressing a nailbed, earlobe or forehead until the skin blanches. Pressure is then released to observe the return of color. Normally, skin color returns to pre-pressure color within two seconds.

7. Interstitial edema
— When the heart is unable to adequately pump blood through its chambers or from the right atrium to the pulmonary artery, the blood backs up or accumulates in the venous system. The backup occurs first in the vena cava then in the venous circulation in the abdomen, particularly in the liver and spleen. The accumulation may extend into the veins of the lower extremities. As the pressure increases within the venous system, intravascular fluid moves out into the interstitial space and is detected as edema.

— In an adult, a considerable amount of fluid can be held in the interstitial space before it is detected as edema. It is not unusual for a weight gain of 5-7 pounds to be attributed to fluid retention. This weight gain converts to 2000-3000 ml of retained fluid within the interstitial space in the most dependent body parts; e.g. ankles or sacrum.

— The degree of interstitial edema is measured by finger indentation to the affected area. The following scale provides consistency among descriptions:

0 = no edema present

+1 = 0 to 1/4-inch indentation which disappears rapidly

+2 = 1/4- to 1/2-inch indentation which disappears within 10-15 seconds

+3 = 1/2- to 1-inch indentation which disappears within 1-2 minutes

+4 = more than 1-inch indentation which lasts longer than 5 minutes

— When the left side of the heart is unable to adequately pump, the phenomenon of edema occurs in the lungs. The intravascular fluid moves from the pulmonary capillaries into the lung interstitial space interfering with gas exchange. If this situation progresses, fluid moves into the alveoli. This fluid is heard by chest auscultation during the respiratory cycle.

— Backup (proximal congestion) of blood from the left side of the heart into the pulmonary vascular system is called pulmonary edema. This condition is often accompanied by a dry, hacking cough. In severe cases, large quantities of frothy, blood-tinged sputum (hemoptysis) may occur.

Supportive Sources of Data

1. Skin color

   — The color of mucous membrane and skin of extremities are indicators of peripheral perfusion when accompanied by one or more primary sources of data.

   — When well-oxygenated hemoglobin is present in the arteriolar microcirculation, the blood appears bright red and the skin surface appears pink. This assessment is more reliable where the capillary network is abundant and near the surface, such as inside the eyelids, gums, nailbeds or earlobes.

   — Other conditions also cause peripheral vasoconstriction and produce color changes similar to poorly oxygenated blood. The physical environment surrounding the person may be cold or the person may be inadequately clothed. Also, the physiological response to stress produces varying degrees of peripheral vasoconstriction.

   — Additional factors affecting gas exchange also produce characteristic changes in skin color. For example, below normal levels of red blood cells or hemoglobin in circulation result in poorly-oxygenated blood. Therefore, a bluish appearance in the periphery (cyanosis) is not a reliable sign of cardiac dysfunction when it is the only observable manifestation.

2. Shortness of breath (dyspnea)

— Circulatory adequacy is closely related to the adequacy of pulmonary gas exchange. Several factors can disrupt cardiopulmonary homeostasis:

• Fluid in lung tissue secondary to a backup of blood from the left side of the heart causes acute shortness of breath.

• An elevated diaphragm secondary to fluid collection in the peritoneal cavity (ascites) impairs ventilatory activity and gas exchange.

• Diminished blood flow from the right ventricle to the pulmonary circulation impairs gas exchange.

— Differentiating between breathlessness at rest and breathlessness with exertion is important. Persons are often not aware of their dyspnea. One apparent clue occurs when these individuals are talking. They frequently interrupt themselves in midsentence to take rapid, shallow breaths.

— Exertional dyspnea is a feeling of breathlessness with certain activities. When accompanied by dry, non-productive cough a cardiac origin is suspected.

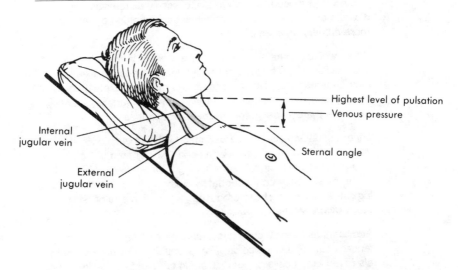

Fig. 3-5. Position of internal and external jugular veins used in measuring venous pressure. W.J. Phipps, B.C. Long, N.F. Woods: Medical-Surgical Nursing: Concepts and Clinical Practices, 5th ed.; St. Louis: Mosby-Year Book, Inc., 1995. Reprinted with permission.

3. Other body system involvement
   - With chronic backup of blood at the entrance to the right side of the heart, venous congestion initially occurs in the vena cava. As blood builds up in the superior vena cava, it can be observed as jugular venous distention (JVD).

   - As the venous congestion builds up in the inferior vena cava, systemic organs become distended. The liver enlarges and is palpable (hepatomegaly).

   - Movement of vascular fluid into the peritoneal cavity increases (ascites) and progressively interferes with digestion and diaphragm movement.

Disrupted Cardiac Function

The interrelationships among impulse transmission, valve effectiveness, pump efficiency and coronary circulation are also affected when dysfunction exists. For example, when a coronary vessel is occluded, electrical impulses are not adequately transmitted across the damaged heart muscle. The pumping capacity of the heart is consequently impaired, and circulation to systemic organs and tissues are affected. Another example of disrupted cardiac function occurs when a streptococcal infection involves the heart muscle (myocardium) and valves. Pumping capacity of the heart is diminished, coronary circulation is impaired and impulse transmission is disrupted.

A variety of clinical situations may disrupt the transmission of impulses in either the atrium or along the ventricular wall. Each abnormal transmission produces a characteristic irregularity or dysrhythmia which can be identified on an EKG recording. While cardiac monitoring is not routine on general medical-surgical nursing units, an understanding of the clinical implications of common dysrhythmias is essential. Dysfunction of other body systems which produce changes in intravascular volume, circulating oxygen or electrolyte levels increase the risk for dysrhythmias.

Electrical Impulse Transmission

1. Normal sequence of transmission
   - As discussed earlier, the normal sequence begins in the SA node and travels to the AV node and then along the neural fibers of the ventricular muscle wall.

   - When the sequence has a normal configuration within a given time interval, it is termed normal sinus rhythm.

   - When normal configurations occur slower than expected, it is termed sinus bradycardia or slow heart rate.

- When normal configurations occur faster than expected, the term sinus tachycardia or fast heart rate is used.

2. Effect of damaged heart muscle on impulse transmission

   - Damaged or scarred myocardium may produce an irregular or delayed sequence. Any change in an established pattern of irregularity may indicate a new problem.

   - A missed segment in the sequence or prolonged transmission time interval is called heart block. The very slow heart rate associated with this dysrhythmia is serious because the heart is incapable of responding when increased cellular metabolic needs require an increased blood supply.

   - An increase in heart rate or cardiac output often may not be met when damaged or scarred myocardium is present.

   - When a seriously slow heart rate persists, an artificial stimulation of impulse transmission or pacemaker may be required to trigger an impulse transmission and a WNL rate.

3. Atrial dysrhythmias

   - Irregularities involving the atrial sequence are associated with extra impulses originating from other locations within the atrium that trigger the ventricular sequence.

   - The heart rate may be markedly increased and may also be irregular because only some of the atrial impulses trigger the ventricular sequence.

   - The most common atrial dysrhythmia is atrial fibrillation. Stimulants such as caffeine, some carbonated soft drinks, allergy medications may produce this clinical problem.

   - If an atrial dysrhythmia persists, blood flow is altered and small blood clots may form. These clots may travel from the left side of the heart and lodge in cerebral arteries (cerebral emboli) or in renal arteries (renal infarction).

4. Ventricular dysrhythmias

   - Ventricular dysrhythmias are more serious as they affect the volume of blood leaving the heart. The cardiac output and circulation to systemic organs and periphery are impaired. Persons with these dysrhythmias are managed in coronary intensive care units (CCU) where they can be continuously monitored.

   - The least serious ventricular dysrhythmia is an occasional premature ventricular contraction (PVC) which often occurs in healthy adults. Caffeine, alcohol intake and stress may contribute to the occurrence.

— The frequency and pattern of PVCs should be well documented as any change may be the forbearer of a more serious and lethal ventricular dysrhythmia. Intravenous Lidocaine
may be administered to control an increasing incidence. However, continuous cardiac monitoring is essential to determine
the response and prompt detection of more serious dysrhythmias. A fast ventricular rate without an associated atrial sequence is termed ventricular tachycardia. A quivering ventricle
(ventricular fibrillation) produces no cardiac output. Both of
these dysrhythmias are cardiac arrest (code) situations and
are the most common cause of sudden cardiac death.

Pump Inefficiency

Problems with the electrical impulse transmission or the circulation to
the heart muscle will affect the efficiency of the pumping capacity of
the heart. When pump efficiency decreases, circulation through the
heart is slowed and congestion develops (congestive heart failure).
The factors of preload, contractility and afterload clarify backup (proximal) and output (distal) effects as they relate to the side of the heart
affected.

1. Preload

   — Preload involves the degree to which the heart can stretch to
   accommodate the blood which remains in the heart after a
   contraction or which fills the ventricle during the resting phase
   of the cardiac cycle (diastole). Backup, buildup and proximal
   effects are terms used to describe the effects of preload on circulation.

   — Fluid overload may increase the volume in the venous system
   and contribute to the problem. The blood first accumulates in
   the chambers of one side of the heart. Progressively the
   blood builds up (backs up) in the anatomical structures proximal to the affected side of the heart.

   — If the circulating volume is less than normal such as with hemorrhage or dehydration, decreased preload is present. The
   heart will attempt to produce an adequate blood flow through
   the heart and vascular system with an adequate cardiac output (CO) by increasing the heart rate. This response explains
   the characteristic signs of shock and hemorrhage: increased
   heart rate and a weak, thready pulse.

   — Changes in preload are associated with specific clinical manifestations of the buildup or backup which can be detected by
   the bedside nurse. Invasive hemodynamic monitoring is utilized when unstable circulatory situations are present. Procedures and equipment like central venous pressures and
   pulmonary capillary pressures provide accurate assessment

data of unstable circulatory conditions in the critical care setting.

2. Contractility
   - The heart muscle contracts in a manner similar to other skele-
     tal muscles. The size, tone and strength of the myocardium in-
     creases in response to the workload required. Therefore,
     ventricular hypertrophy refers to the enlarged muscle wall of
     the lower chamber of the heart.

   - If the heart muscle is damaged (cardiomyopathy) or when a
     sudden, intense or sustained metabolic need is present, the
     heart muscle may not be physically fit. The ability of the heart
     to produce sufficient contractility may not be possible and the
     heart will begin to fail.

   - Decreased contractility may lead to decreased emptying of the
     heart chambers and subsequent increasing preload. De-
     creased contractility also results in a decreased flow of blood
     out of the heart and decreased perfusion.

   - The presence of cool extremities and cyanotic or mottled skin
     color are suggestive of decreased contractility and impaired pe-
     ripheral circulation. Further assessment is required to deter-
     mine the cause of these symptoms.

3. Afterload
   - Afterload refers to the resistance against which the heart must
     pump. The major resistance is caused by narrowing or ob-
     structed arterial vessels. Atherosclerotic plaques are the most
     common cause which lead to systemic hypertension and vaso-
     constriction.

   - Output and distal effects are terms used to describe the blood
     flow related to afterload problems and circulatory conse-
     quences to systemic body organs and the periphery.

   - Markedly and sustained elevated systolic pressures may dam-
     age or rupture weakened arteries (aneurysms, hemorrhage).
     Markedly and sustained diastolic pressures damage the micro-
     circulation in major organs and impair their physiological func-
     tioning (retinal hemorrhage, impaired renal function).

   - Sustained increased afterload will eventually affect contractility
     and lead to increased preload. There is a progressive back
     up proximal to cause of the afterload.

Measures to Improve Circulatory Efficiency

Measures to improve circulatory efficiency focus on decreasing the preload and afterload and improving the contractility of the heart. In most situations, medical, non-surgical interventions are initiated first.

1. Medications

    — Five major categories of medications are commonly prescribed to improve circulatory efficiency: antihypertensives, diuretics, glycosides, antiarrhythmics, anticoagulants.

        NOTE: Only an introduction to the major effects related to circulatory improvement is presented in this section. The topic of nursing implications of pharmacological management is extensive, therefore, additional reading from other sources is recommended.

    — Control of the underlying pathophysiological problem, hypertension, is the first approach to pharmacological intervention. Some medications act directly to lower the serum level of cholesterol in an attempt to delay the development of atherosclerotic plaques. Zocar (simvastatin) is one medication prescribed to lower serum cholesterol levels. The safest method is to reduce the total dietary fat intake.

    — When placque formation has progressed to the point of reducing the lumen (opening) of arteries, then control of hypertension is the focus. Various antihypertensive medications are available to modify the systemic vascular resistance (SVR) by a variety of physiological mechanisms. The goal of hypertensive pharmacological management is to reduce the blood pressure with minimal side effects.

    — Peripheral vasodilators (nitrates, nitroglycerine) relax the smooth muscles of the arteries. Some anti-hypertensive agents block a segment in the chemical sequence leading to vasoconstriction (beta blockers, calcium channel blockers). Other agents interfere with the renin-angiotensin cycle (ACE inhibitors). Most anti-hypertensives are prescribed in combinations with another medication.

    — Diuretic medications (Lasix/furosemide, Maxide/spironolactone) are often prescribed in combination with antihypertensives to lower blood pressure. Diuretics decrease the amount of fluid in circulation by increasing fluid excretion from the kidneys. Pooled interstitial fluid then moves into the vascular compartment and is excreted. Cardiac workload decreases when normal amounts of fluid are located in the vascular and interstitial compartments.

- Cardiac glycosides (digitalis, Lanoxin, Digitoxin) are commonly prescribed to improve the pumping capacity of the heart. This effect is accomplished by decreasing the heart rate and increasing the force of cardiac muscle contraction. The desired effect can be exaggerated when there is a significant loss of potassium secondary to diuretic therapy.

- Less serious dysrhythmias are controlled by agents that block the extra impulse transmissions (Procardia/nifedipine, Inderal/propranolol). Avoiding foods and liquids with caffeine also minimize the occurrence of irregular impulse transmissions.

- Anticoagulant therapy is prescribed to minimize the formation or extension of an existing blood clot. Acute situations are treated by intermittent injection or continuous intravenous infusion of heparin by a dosage that is adjusted or titrated by the serial laboratory testing of the clotting response, the partial thromboplastin time or PTT. Maintenance dosage of oral anticoagulants (Coumadin) minimize clot recurrence which is monitored by prothrombin time (PT).

- Thrombolytic agents (streptokinase, TPA) are used to dissolve an established blood clot and restore vessel patency. This acute treatment can be initiated within the first few hours following an occluded coronary artery or myocardial infarction. It is usually administered in a CCU or a unit where continuous cardiac monitoring is available. Ventricular dysrhythmias and cardiac instability may occur with this therapy.

- With the use of anticoagulant or anti-thrombolytic therapy, measures to prevent bleeding are essential. Bleeding may occur from mucous membrane, injection sites or along the gastrointestinal tract.

2. Oxygen therapy

- Oxygen therapy is administered to persons with circulatory problems to prevent or minimize the consequences of tissue hypoxia. For persons with myocardial damage, oxygen may correct some dysrhythmias, such as premature ventricular contractions (PVCs).

- When a concurrent chronic respiratory problem is present, oxygen must be administered cautiously.

3. Measures to decrease cardiac workload

- When the heart must pump harder or faster, there is an increased cardiac workload. A decrease in physical activity or rest is the primary intervention to decrease the workload. This goal is sometimes difficult to accomplish as the person experiencing an acute cardiac episode is very anxious and restless.

The cycle of anxiety, physiological stress, increased cardiac activity and cardiac pain are managed by sedatives and analgesics.

— Vasoconstriction is one cause of systemic vascular resistance (SVR) and increased afterload. An elevated blood pressure is an indicator of the degree of resistance against which the heart must pump.

— Pain relief and antihypertensive agents minimize the adverse effects of an acute cardiac episode. During an acute cardiac crisis, large dosages of Demerol or morphine are prescribed. At this point in the management and care, pain relief and decrease of cardiac workload have a higher priority than the possibility of addiction.

— Stress management and biofeedback are effective for some persons for long-term control of situations which may precipitate hypertensive crisis and chest pain.

— When there is an insufficient number of oxygen carriers (red blood cells and hemoglobin), the heart works harder to circulate the available blood faster. The resultant tachycardia and fatigability are an indication of this compensatory response.

— Morphine and nitroglycerine may also be used for their vasodilating effects.

— With the relaxation of pulmonary vessels, preload may be decreased. With arterial relaxation, systemic vascular resistence (SVR) and afterload are decreased.

4. Measures to decrease cellular metabolism
    — Optimally, there is a balance between an adequate supply of oxygen and cellular need. When certain pathophysiological conditions occur at the cellular level and the need for oxygen increases, an imbalance develops.

    — Oxygen consumption can increase from 30-100% with an infection, trauma or a serious burn. If the heart is healthy, the cardiac rate and output increases to meet the cellular need. However, when the heart is not physically fit or damaged, it cannot sufficiently respond, and a deficit occurs.

    — Measures to maintain normal body temperature and to create a minimally stimulating environment will facilitate physiological functioning within normal levels.

    — Spacing hygienic and therapeutic care activities to allow for rest periods will restore the balance between oxygen supply and cellular demand. Evaluation of an individual's ability to tolerate these activities is determined by assessing tissue perfusion. A change in cardiac activity (blood pressure, pulse) or change in agitation or restlessness combined with changes in skin color may indicate that cellular consumption is beyond the capacity of the heart and lungs to deliver an adequate oxygen supply.

5. Surgical interventions
   — Valve replacement is indicated for the individual with valve dysfunction that is impairing perfusion and affecting quality of life. While any valve may be damaged, the mitral valve, which is located between the left atrium and left ventricle, is the most commonly involved and most often replaced.

   — Revascularization

   • Coronary artery by-pass (CAB) involves the surgical placement of segments of the saphenous vein or mammary artery to segments of the coronary artery to circumvent localized vessel blockage. This common procedure improves the quality of life for individuals with coronary artery disease.

   • Percutaneous transluminal coronary angioplasty (PTCA) offers another method for reopening blocked coronary arteries. This less invasive procedure involves the use of a balloon catheter that is inserted into the affected coronary artery to compress a localized atherosclerotic placque against the arterial wall.

   • An endarterectomy is the surgical removal of localized atherosclerotic plaques usually from a carotid artery to improve the circulation to the brain.

   • A thrombectomy is the surgical removal of an established blood clot from a major artery or vein. Fibrinolytic agents (streptokinase, urokinase) may be used to dissolve an acute peripheral thrombus. Tissue-type plasminogen activator (TPA) is another thrombolytic agent used following an acute myocardial infarction. Inferior vena cava filters or umbrellas may be surgically inserted to entrap fragments from recurrent clots in an extremity from traveling and lodging in the pulmonary vasculature (pulmonary emboli).

SECTION 3: CLINICAL EXAMPLES OF CARDIAC DYSFUNCTION

Atherosclerosis

Arteriosclerosis is a chronic disease of arteries characterized by abnormal thickening and hardening of the vessel wall. The smooth muscle of the vessel is replaced with fibrous tissue. Progressively the vessel loses its ability to change the size of the inner opening (diameter).

Atherosclerosis is a form of arteriosclerosis. Initially fatty (cholesterol) deposits occur in the inner layer of the vessel. These deposits and fibrous buildup progressively involve the muscle layer of the vessel and gradually the vessel opening becomes narrowed. The plaque buildup increases the resistance to blood flow resulting in hypertension and diminished circulation to all body organs. The delivery of an adequate supply of oxygenated blood and nutrients for cellular metabolism is impaired.

The inner most layer of the affected artery becomes irregular which causes an aggregation of red blood cells at the involved sites. Thromboses (blood clots) may develop and occlude the vessel. This is the pathophysiology of a "heart attack" or myocardial infarction, cerebral vascular accident (CVA or stroke) and peripehral arterial insufficiency.

As the plaque formation progressively invades the arterial muscle, the wall of the artery may become thin and weakened. As the blood pressure increases, these thinned areas may bulge forming an aneurysm. Episodes of elevated blood pressure may cause an aneurysm to rupture and cause a life-threatening hemorrhage. The aorta and cerebral arteries are the common sites of this complication. Successful surgical repair of an aneurysm is possible if diagnosed before rupture has occurred.

While the atherosclerotic process occurs in all arteries, this section will focus on the clinical manifestations and consequences related to coronary and major artery dysfunction. Cerebral consequences resulting in a cerebral vascular accident (CVA) are discussed in Unit 1: Neurological Dysfunction.

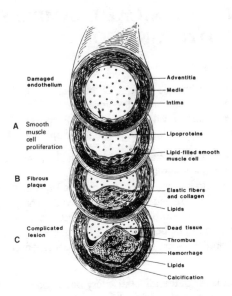

Fig. 3-6. The development in the progression of atherosclerosis include: (A) smooth muscle cell proliferation, which creates (B) a raised fibrous plaque and (C) a complicated lesion. From S.M. Lewis, I.C. Collier: Medical-Surgical Nursing: Assessment and Management of Clinical Problems, 4th ed.; St. Louis: Mosby-Year Book, Inc., 1995. Reprinted with permisision.

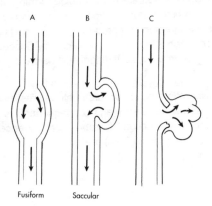

Fig. 3-7. Aneurysm types: (A) true fusiform aneurysm; (B) true saccular aneurysm; (C) false aneurysm. From S.A. Price, L.M. Wilson: Pathophysiology: Clinical Concepts of Disease Processes, 4th ed.; St. Louis: Mosby-Year Book, Inc., 1992. Reprinted with permission.

Hypertension

Hypertension (HTN) is defined as a persistent systolic blood pressure greater than 140 mm Hg and/or a persistent diastolic blood pressure greater than 90 mm Hg. Elevations in blood pressure occur gradually or suddenly. A gradual rise may be asymptomatic as the functioning of the body systems progressively adjusts and accommodates to the elevation. A sudden rise, on the other hand, produces acute symptoms and sudden impairment of body system functioning.

1. Chronic hypertension will affect the physiological functioning of other body systems. For example, kidney function will progressively become impaired and can lead to chronic renal insufficiency and eventually chronic renal failure (CRF).

2. Chronic hypertension may cause small arterioles to rupture. When this occurs in the retina of the eye, blindness may result.

3. Primary (essential, idiopathic) hypertension has no identifiable medical cause. Other forms of hypertension develop subsequent to a specific physiological cause, e.g. renal vascular narrowing, certain drugs, organ dysfunction, tumors or pregnancy. Malignant hypertension refers to an abrupt onset and accelerated course which may cause rapid deterioration of the individual's condition.

4. Subtle signs of progressive hypertension include: headaches especially upon rising in the morning, blurred vision, unsteadiness, or spontaneous nosebleeds (epistaxis).

5. Medication and diet therapy are the primary methods of control to achieve BP below 140/90. Initially blood pressure control is attempted with nonpharmacological therapy; e.g. sodium and alcohol restriction, weight control, regular physical activity and cessation of cigarette smoking.

   — If hypertension persists, a diuretic (Lasix/furosemide, Maxide/spironolactone,), beta blocker (Aldomet/methyldopa, Inderal/propranolol, Lopressor/metoprolol), calcium antagonist (Cardizem/deltiazem, Procardia/nifedipine), or ACE inhibitor (Capoten/captopril) is prescribed.

   — If hypertension persists, the dosage is increased or a substitution is made.

   — If hypertension persists, a second category of antihypertensive medication is also prescribed.

   — If hypertension persists and an emergency state exists, intravenous drip of nitroprusside (Nipride) may be administered because of its immediate vasodilating action.

6. When diuretics are utilized, periodic assessments of serum potassium levels are warranted. With the increased excretion of fluid and sodium, potassium is also excreted. As potassium is not stored, daily requirements must be met. Unless concurrent renal dysfunction is present, potassium supplements may be required (K-LOR, potassium chloride/KCL).

7. Noncompliance is a major reason for inadequate HTN control. One reason is that as the blood pressure is restored within normal limits, related symptoms diminish and the individual is unaware of the continuing subtle damage to other organs. A second factor is the occurrence of unpleasant side effects associated with some anti-hypertensive agents. Multiple medications to be taken at varying times is often problematic for the elderly and frequently dosages are missed. Systematic follow-up of persons, their response to prescribed therapies and control of side effects increases compliance.

Ischemic Heart Disease

This is a progressive condition that results from atherosclerosis and is commonly associated with hypertension and diabetes mellitus. There is a progressive impairment of the arterial perfusion through the coronary arteries supplying the heart muscle (myocardium). When the vessel narrowing cannot deliver an adequate supply of oxygenated blood and nutrients needed for cardiac activity, acute ischemic clinical manifestations occur (angina). When the vessel becomes occluded and a thrombosis develops, the subsequent tissue hypoxia distal to the occlusion results in cellular damage (ischemia) and cell death (infarction) of the muscle wall of the heart. The transmission of electrical impulses is disrupted in the affected area and subsequently the contractility of the heart is impaired. Depending upon the extent of damage, perfusion to other parts of the body is affected which may lead to a state of cardiogenic shock.

Angina

1. Coronary Artery Disease (CAD) is the most common example of ischemic heart disease. The most characteristic symptom of CAD is chest pain (angina) which is caused by a temporary inadequate blood supply to the heart muscle. It often occurs during exercise or physical activity and subsides with rest. It may also occur during periods of decreased circulation or hypotension.

   — Interventions to delay the progression of CAD:

      • Diet low in cholesterol, sodium, triglycerides, calories and caffeine-free foods and liquids.

- Relaxation and stress management techniques.

- Reduction and control of risk behaviors especially cigarette smoking.

- Planned, regular exercise program to increase the physical fitness of the heart and develop collateral circulation around affected vessels.

- Control of hypertension, diabetes mellitus, obesity.

2. "Angina" chest pain is described as a pressure or agonizing substernal pain that radiates down one or both arms. It may also be felt in the neck, cheeks and teeth. It may be misinterpreted by the individual as acute indigestion, especially if it occurs after eating a heavy meal. Exposure to cold temperatures may precipitate angina symptoms.

   — An elderly person may not experience typical pain because of changes in neuroreceptors. Weakness or fainting are more characteristic.

3. An EKG and cardiac enzymes (CPK, LDH) are usually normal as there is no permanent tissue damage.

4. Stress test or treadmill exercise test with continuous cardiac monitoring will determine the amount of exercise that causes angina and degree of ischemia. 24-hour ambulatory monitoring also can identify ischemia-induced changes in impulse transmission.

5. Coronary arteriography via cardiac catheterization provides the definitive diagnosis. An angioplasty (PTCA) may be performed to improve the coronary blood flow at the time of the catheterization. A tiny balloon is inflated at the end of the catheter to compress the plaque material against the vessel wall. If the coronary perfusion is not improved, the surgical intervention or revascularization by a coronary artery by-pass graft (CABG) is considered. Care of individuals experiencing these interventions are usually cared for on a coronary care unit (CCU) as there is a risk for acute cardiac dysrhythmias.

6. Angina pain may be managed by patient self-medication using nitroglycerine tablets. This medication is administered sublingually and can be repeated three times every five minutes. The individual should remain recumbent during administration as hypotension and headaches are common side effects. The individual should be advised that if pain relief does not occur with the recommended administration, the physician or medical provider should be notified.

— This medication is unstable and should be kept in a securely-capped dark glass container (not metal or plastic pillboxes). It is deactivated by heat, moisture, air, light and time. The prescription should be renewed every 6 months.

— Normally, a dosage will produce a burning sensation under the tongue and often a fullness or throbbing in the head. Side effects include flushing, throbbing headache, hypotension and tachycardia.

— Nitroglycerine tablets may be taken prophylactically to avoid angina pain that may occur with certain physical activities, e.g. stair climbing, sexual intercourse.

7. Care during an angina attack and during hospitalization follows a similar pattern. In addition to the previously stated interventions, the heart rate and blood pressure should be monitored. Identification and reporting of an irregularity in the heart rate or a decrease of 20 mmHg in the systolic blood pressure from an established baseline are important in the early intervention of a possible complication.

8. The administration of oxygen as prescribed during an attack will ensure an adequate supply of oxygenated blood to the myocardium and may minimize the occurrence of hypoxic dysrhythmias.

Acute Myocardial Infarction (MI or "heart attack")

If a condition which causes ischemia to the myocardium persists, permanent damage to cardiac tissue occurs. Individuals experiencing an acute MI are usually treated on a coronary care unit where continuous cardiac monitoring is available. However, it is necessary for the general medical-surgical nurse to recognize the characteristics of an acute MI because this condition may occur to an individual who has been hospitalized for a non-cardiac condition.

1. Acute myocardial chest pain is characterized by a sudden and usually severe onset of chest pain which is not relieved by rest or any intervention except the administration of narcotics, such as morphine. The pain usually radiates to the left arm and is described as a crushing or vise-like pain which surrounds the chest. It may increase steadily in severity until it becomes almost unbearable.

— Often among the elderly, the pain is atypical; e.g. jaw pain or fainting. Concurrent peripheral vascular resistance and HTN mask the symptoms of impaired coronary perfusion until tissue damage had occurred.

— The individual with acute chest pain should be treated as having an MI until it has been ruled out and another cause of the chest pain has been identified.

2. If the pumping capacity of the heart is affected, there will be varying accompanying clinical manifestations of impaired perfusion to other body parts. The signs of shock appear: pallor with diaphoresis; fall in blood pressure; weak, irregular or rapid pulse rate, increased anxiety and restlessness.

3. If an acute MI is suspected the following data should be obtained for reporting to the physician:

   — Description of the chest pain.

   — Measures initiated to relieve the pain and the response.

   — Supporting assessment data: current and baseline vital signs.

4. If an acute MI is suspected, the bedside nurse could anticipate the following orders:

   — Serum blood chemistry analysis with cardiac enzymes (CPK and LDH). These enzymes are elevated in a characteristic pattern when myocardial damaged has occurred.

   — 12 lead EKG to identify the location and extent of tissue damage.

   — Bedrest in semi-Fowler's position to conserve cardiac workload.

   — Oxygen by nasal cannula, usually 2-6 L/minute is adjusted based on oxygen saturation measurement and concurrent chronic lung disease.

   — Complete blood count (CBC) which usually reveals leukocytosis secondary to the inflammatory response.

   — Relief of the acute pain with IV morphine sulfate or nitroglycerine by IV drip.

5. The individual is usually transferred to a coronary care unit where continuous cardiac monitoring is available. The majority of MI deaths during hospitalization occur within the first 2 hours of onset of chest pain and are due to ventricular dysrhythmias. Therefore, the prevention, identification and early treatment of these dysrhythmias are essential. It is estimated that the incidence of dysrhythmias after an acute MI is 90%.

6. Medical reperfusion with thrombolytic therapy using streptokinase or tissue plasminogen activator (TPA) can be initiated within the first few hours following an acute MI. This intervention breaks down, or lyses, the fibrin clot before it is established. Whereas, anticoagulant therapy minimizes the recurrence or extension of an existing thrombus.

7. It is estimated that 50% of all myocardial infarctions are uncompl-
    icated with no evidence of severe dysrhythmias, congestive heart
    failure or shock. Most individuals are discharged from the hospital
    within 7-10 days.

8. When the individual is symptom-free, active cardiac rehabilitation is
    provided. The goals of the four phase program are to extend and
    improve the quality of life so the individual can return to a normal
    or near-normal life style.

    —   Phase I begins in CCU with an assessment of the individual's
        understanding of his condition and what is happening. Physi-
        cal conditioning includes range of motion for the arms and pro-
        gressive activity.

    —   Phase II occurs during the remainder of hospitalization. The
        focus is positively directed on what the individual will be able
        to do with some modification after discharge. Understanding
        the disease and therapies is essential for compliance after dis-
        charge. Physical conditioning includes walking and some stair
        climbing with portable (holter) monitoring.

    —   Phase III begins after discharge and continues during conva-
        lescence with supervised increments in physical activity and
        the goal of returning to work or to pre-MI activities. Physical
        conditioning includes more vigorous walking at regular inter-
        vals.

    —   Phase IV focuses on long term conditioning and cardiovascu-
        lar stability. Physical conditioning now includes jogging.

Congestive Heart Failure (CHF)

Heart failure is a state in which the heart is no longer able to pump
sufficient quantities of oxygenated blood and nutrients for cellular metabolism to the tissues. This failure may be an acute condition resulting from a myocardial infarction or it may develop subtly and
progressively. Either or both sides of the heart may be affected.

Problems with the electrical impulse transmission, anatomical structures or circulation to the heart muscle affect the efficiency of the
pumping capacity of the heart. When pumping efficiency decreases,
circulation through the heart is slowed and congestion develops (congestive heart failure). The factors of preload, contractility and
afterload clarify backup (proximal) and output (distal) effects as they relate to the side of the heart affected.

Focused Bedside Cardiac Assessment

The following is a guideline of data that would be expected from a head-to-toe assessment of an individual with an acute uncomplicated MI. No other pathophysiological problem involving other body systems is included.

* **General appearance:** Appears in acute distress; sitting upright; diaphoretic; pale. Complains of sharp, continuous chest pain that radiates down the left arm, into jaw, or through to back.

* **Level of consciousness:** Restless; oriented to person, place and time.

* **Head and neck:** Perspiration on the forehead. While sitting in semi-Fowler's position of 30' elevation, no jugular vein distention noted.

* **Cardiac status:** Difficulty hearing heart sounds because of pulmonary crackles. Apical heart rate is 90 and irregular without a pattern. Blood pressure is 107/70; baseline BP is 124/70. **NOTE:** The heart rate may also be markedly slow indicating the possibility of a heart block.

* **Respiratory status:** Crackles auscultated in lower lung fields since the onset of chest pain. They were not present on earlier assessment. Respiratory rate is 24/minute without any apparent difficulty. No cough noted.

* **Abdomen:** Soft with hypoactive bowel sounds. No pain on palpation. Liver borders nonpalpatable.

* **Urinary elimination:** Voided 150 ml in the last hour. Appeared clear and yellow. Reagent strips are negative for glucose, ketones and blood.

* **Extremities:** Pedal pulses are faint and palpable in both feet. Capillary refill is less than 2 seconds in all extremities. Hands and feet feel cold with mild cyanosis of the nailbeds. Skin is damp with perspiration.

* When the person is turned on their side, the nurse assesses that no sacral edema is present. Posterior breath sounds reveal coarse crackles in both lower lung fields.

If additional data is observed, a more detailed assessment of the involved system is required. Additional areas of physiological dysfunction may be present and confound the present circulatory problem.

1. Left-sided heart failure

   — Failure of the left side of the heart to adequately pump blood from its chambers out into the general circulation results in impaired delivery of oxygenated blood and nutrients to the cells of the body. The distal consequences of this output problem is a state of cardiogenic shock.

— The proximal consequences of blood not adequately flowing through the left chambers results in backup or congestion in the lungs. The increased pressure within the pulmonary veins in the lungs causes intravascular fluid to move into the lung tissue (pulmonary interstitial edema). As the pressure continues, fluid moves into the alveoli (pulmonary edema).

— Dyspnea results from the accumulation of fluid in the alveoli. Impaired gas exchange and associated restlessness are precipitated by minimal physical activity.

• Orthopnea refers to increased difficulty breathing when the individual lies flat. Therefore, the person must be propped upright with pillows or sit in a chair to sleep.

• Paroxysmal nocturnal dyspnea (PND) occurs primarily at night. These individuals sit in a chair for long periods of time during the day allowing relatively large amounts of fluid to accumulate in dependent body parts. When the individual returns to bed in a recumbent position, the fluid from the lower extremities returns to the venous system and circulation. This increase in intravascular volume is greater than the ability of the heart to pump the blood effectively through the chambers; thus, backup or congestion rapidly develops in the lungs causing dyspnea.

— This pulmonary fluid can be heard on auscultation as wheezes, crackles or rhonchi. Often the person also experiences a dry, hacking cough. More advanced symptoms include frothy, blood tinged sputum (hemoptysis) and respiratory failure.

— As this condition may develop rapidly, early detection by the bedside nurse is essential. The person is usually transferred to a critical care unit where their vital signs and hemodynamic state can be continuously monitored.

2. Right-sided heart failure

— As the blood from the right side of the heart is pumped to the lungs where gas exchange occurs, the distal consequences are observed as decreased cardiac output and impaired perfusion to the periphery.

— The proximal consequences of the blood not adequately flowing through the right chambers of the heart results in back up or congestion in the vena cava at the entrance to the right atrium. As the blood continues to back up in the venous system, abdominal organs become distended with accumulated blood. Intravascular fluid moves into the peritoneal cavity (ascites). Further backup leads to congested veins in the legs and the development of dependent edema.

— Congestion of blood in the liver may cause enlargement (hepatomegaly) and the liver may be palpated below the lower right rib cage. An enlarged liver can also elevate the diaphragm and further compromise ventilatory activity and gas exchange.

— An infection is a common precipitating factor for an acute episode of right-sided CHF. The metabolic needs during an infection are increased and may be beyond the capability of the heart to deliver the required oxygen and nutrients. For example, in the elderly, an upper respiratory tract infection may quickly lead to pneumonia. The respiratory symptoms of developing pneumonia often closely mimic the congestive symptoms of heart failure and may progress unnoticed and untreated until an acute circulatory situation exists.

— Progressive intolerance to physical activity and increasing fatigability are related to decreased cardiac contractility. Therefore, activities of daily living (ADL) should be paced to minimize shortness of breath. Concurrent anemia may further exaggerate fatigability and activity intolerance.

— Intravascular fluid overload may develop gradually and go unnoticed. Cues to the presence of fluid overload include:

  • Gradual elevation in the blood pressure over baseline.

  • Progressive development of dependent edema is especially noticeable in the morning. In addition, the hands feel full/"fat" and rings are tight, especially in the morning.

  • Nocturia will develop as a compensatory response to decreased cardiac workload while sleeping. During physiological rest the excess fluid moves from the interstitial space into the intravascular compartment and then is excreted at frequent intervals.

  • Progressive intolerance to lying flat without shortness of breath. The size or number of pillows used to permit sleep increases.

  • Gradual weight gain not associated with increased caloric intake.

3. Treatment modalities

  — Diuretics to decrease the intravascular volume in circulation

  — Cardiotonics to increase the cardiac contractility

  — Decreased sodium intake to minimize fluid retention

  — Potassium supplement to minimize the loss from diuretic therapy

Focused Bedside Assessment

The following is a guideline of data that would be expected from a head-to-toe assessment of an individual admitted with an acute exascerbation of right-sided congestive heart failure. No other pathophysiological problems involving other body system dysfunction unrelated to congestive heart failure is included.

* **General appearance:** Tired and weak; general malaise; poor appetite.

* **Level of consciousness:** If gas exchange is impaired, signs of hypoxia may be present: restlessness, confusion; or signs of hypercapnia may be present: lethargy.

* **Head and neck:** Jugular veins may be full to distended.

* **Cardiac status:** Heart rate may be slowed, irregular, weak or increased depending upon the underlying cardiac dysfunction. Due to increased lungs sounds and an enlarged heart, it may be difficult to hear the heart sounds and any abnormalities. Having the individual lie on their left side often increases auscultation and clarity of heart sounds. Extra heart sounds that mimic a "gallop" may be heard.

* **Respiratory status:** Increased adventious sounds are expected. Establishing a baseline for future comparison is essential. Orthopnea and labored breathing may also be evident.

* **Abdomen:** Ascites and hepatomegaly may be present if CHF is a long standing clinical problem. Establishing a baseline of daily weights and urinary output is essential for future comparison.

* **Urinary elimination:** Urinary patterns may be irregular due to changes in circulating volume during a 24-hour period. The amount and nature of urine should be established. Often an underlying urinary tract infection or prostatic hypertrophy may be the precipitating etiology for an acute episode of congestive heart failure.

* **Extremities:** Dependent edema is a common manifestation. Determine the degree of pitting. Peripheral pulses are present but may be weak or irregular.

* When the individual is turned on their side, the nurse would expect to find: Congestion in all lung fields consistent with the anterior findings. If the individual had been in bed, dependent edema may be noted in the sacral area.

If additional data is observed, a more detailed assessment of the involved system is required. Additional areas of physiological dysfunction may be present and confound the present circulatory problem.

— Antihypertensive agents decrease the vascular resistance against which the heart must pump

Valvular Problems

Infection and inflammation may affect the heart muscle (carditis), the inner layer of the heart (endocarditis) or the valves. The most common infectious process of the heart results from a streptococcal infection ("strep throat"). The sequela of infection, systemic involvement and rheumatic heart disease may cause permanent cardiac damage and inefficient pump capacity. Clinical manifestations may be sudden and associated with the acute infection, or manifestations of heart failure may develop later in life when increased cardiac workload is required.

1. Rheumatic carditis and cardiomyopathy

    This cardiac condition is directly attributed to rheumatic fever, a systemic disease caused by a streptococcal infection. The heart or kidneys may be affected by the secondary inflammatory response. Initially, the myocardium becomes weakened and loses its contractile power.

    −   In most cases, the heart heals with little residual impairment. Occasionally, later in life when a non-cardiac state requires increased cardiac workload, the myocardium may not be able to sustain prolonged increased activity. Signs of heart failure may develop.

    −   Sometimes the infectious process may lead to scarring of tendons that control the movement of the valve, especially in the left heart (mitral stenosis). The aortic and tricuspid valves may be affected but less frequently. The mitral valve is located between the left atrium and left ventricle.

    −   As the valves may not close completely when the ventricle contracts, blood flows back into the atrium (valve insufficiency or regurgitation). When the aortic valve does not completely close following a heart beat, the blood flows back into the left ventricle (aortic insufficiency or regurgitation)

    −   Back up in the left side of the heart quickly leads to pulmonary congestion (pulmonary edema). Prompt recognition of symptoms and initiation of treatment are required to relieve the fluid overload and to improve the contractility of the heart.

2. Infective endocarditis

    −   Persons with cardiac valve disease are at risk for two additional complications due to the irregularity of the inside surface of the heart and slowed circulation: (1) circulating bacteria may grow on the damaged valves and (2) blood clots may form.

- General manifestations may resemble influenza with vague complaints of malaise, cough, joint pain and intermittent fever. Small hemorrhagic streaks are often noted under fingernails and toenails, or petechiae may be noted on the chest.

- Cardiac involvement reveals heart murmurs, cardiomegaly or evidence of congestive failure.

- Fragments of bacterial growth or clots may break away from the infected area. They leave the left side of the heart and are carried to other parts of the body (emboli). As 20% of the blood is pumped to the brain and another 15-20% is pumped into the kidneys, emboli are likely to be carried to these major organs and obstruct arteries (cerebral artery occlusion or renal infarction).

- Long-term antibiotic therapy is prescribed for high risk persons to minimize the infectious sequence. Persons who have had valve replacement, previous endocarditis episodes, or cardiac malformations are at risk. Any invasive procedure that is associated with transient bacteremia may cause the bacteria to lodge in damaged, irregular valves.

- Surgical replacement of damaged valves is now successful even in older adults.

SECTION 4: PERIPHERAL VASCULAR DYSFUNCTION

Overview of Disrupted Vascular Function

All peripheral vascular disorders are characterized by disturbances in the blood flow through the peripheral vessels. This circulatory impairment leads to disturbances in cellular metabolism. When the arterial vessels are involved, adequate supplies of oxygen and nutrients are not delivered to the microcirculation (capillaries) and eventually the cells. When the venous or lymphatic structures are involved, there is an accumulation of the end products of cellular metabolism (lactic and pyruvic acids) and fluid. The localized acidosis and fluid stasis leads to further cellular injury.

Atherosclerosis and advanced diabetes mellitus are the primary causes of arterial impairment. Incompetent venous valves (varicose veins) and thrombophlebitis are the common causes of venous impairment. Prompt care of the underlying causes and excellent foot care will prevent further complications. Skin breakdown from impaired peripheral circulation may lead to prolonged and recurrent hospitalizations, increased morbidity, vascular by-pass surgery and possible amputation. Preventive measures are easier to implement than corrective ones.

Assessment of Peripheral Perfusion

Persons with peripheral vascular dysfunction usually experience symptoms of pain, cramps, swelling and changes in skin temperature of the affected extremity. Concurrent medical problems such as diabetes mellitus and hypertension are also present, which must be considered in the assessment and planning of care.

1. Characteristics of arterial and venous problems

   — When arterial circulation cannot deliver oxygenated blood to a distal location, that portion of the body appears pale or cyanotic and feels cool. The subsequent tissue hypoxia and ischemia causes varying degrees of pain. Peripheral pulses are diminished or absent.

   — When venous return to the heart is impaired, deoxygenated blood pools in the affected area. A feeling of fullness and warmth with a dark red to purple appearance of the skin is characteristic. The associated venous congestion leads to the development of edema in the tissues dependent and proximal to the venous obstruction. Peripheral pulses are usually unaffected.

2. Pain

   — Intermittent claudication refers to ischemia in the peripheral arterial system. The pathophysiology and clinical manifestations are similar to the consequences of atherosclerosis in the coronary arteries leading to angina. With physical activity such as walking, the person experiences increasing muscular pain in an extremity associated with muscular weakness, muscle aching or cramping and sometimes numbness. The severity of these symptoms diminishes with rest and increases with exertion.

   — As the arterial occlusion progresses, the pain increases in severity and lasts longer with rest. It eventually occurs without activity and is often worse at night. Shooting sensations (lancinating pain) to the feet and toes may occur. It is not relieved by rest and is usually aggravated by elevating the affected part.

3. Peripheral pulses
    — Pulses may be diminished or absent with arterial insufficiency
      and are usually unaffected with venous insufficiency. As inter-
      stitial edema is often present with venous impairment, locating
      a pulse may be difficult and a doppler may be needed.

    — Peripheral pulses can be palpated at sites where major arter-
      ies are near the surface of the skin which include: carotid, bra-
      chial, radial, ulnar, femoral, popliteal, posterior tibial and
      dorsalis pedis.

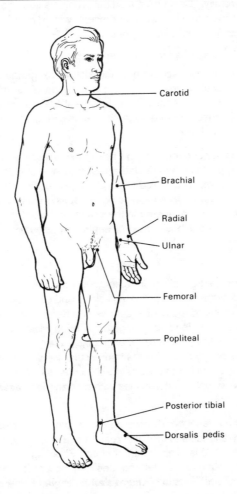

— Carotid

— Brachial

— Radial

— Ulnar

— Femoral

— Popliteal

— Posterior tibial

— Dorsalis pedis

Fig. 3-8. Peripheral pulses. Form S.M. Lewis, I.C. Collier: Medical-Surgical Nursing:
Assessment and Management of Clinical Problems, 4th ed.; St. Louis: Mosby-Year Book,
Inc., 1995. Reprinted with permission.

- The pressure or volume of the pulse is described by the following terms: normal, bounding, thready or absent.

A numerical scale may also be used:

0 =   absent

1+ =   barely palpable

2+ =   decreased

3+ =   full (normal)

4+ =   bounding

4. Capillary refill

- With normal cardiac function and adequate microcirculation, normal response to compression of a nailbed or tissue ensures capillary refill in less than two seconds. Skin and environmental temperatures affect or mask capillary refill times.

5. Dependent edema

- Interstitial edema is often associated with venous insufficiency due to the venous congestion. It may be pitting and is often more apparent at the end of the day than in the morning. The severity is often minimized by elevating the affected extremity to facilitate venous return to the heart.

- During an acute episode, daily measurement of the circumference of the affected extremity provide comparative data about status of the inflammatory process.

Diagnostic Measures

1. Homan's sign is positive when the foot is flexed upward (dorsiflexed) and sharp pain is felt in the calf of the leg and is indicative of an acute venous inflammation (phlebitis).

2. Graded leg raising is a systematic assessment of arterial perfusion of the lower extremities and feet. Insufficiency is associated with increased grayish pallor of the feet when elevated 60 degrees. Usually the local discomfort or pain is increased with a positive finding.

3. Allen test is an assessment of arterial perfusion to the hands. When the radial artery (radial pulse site) is compressed and the hand is clenched, there is pallor of the hand. When the hand is unclenched and the ulnar artery no longer compressed, the hand becomes pink, indicating that the ulnar artery is patent. If the pallor persists as long as the radial artery is compressed, ulnar artery occlusion is probable.

4. Angiography and venography are more definitive tests to identify the exact location of an occlusion and the presence of collateral circulation.

Measures to Improve Peripheral Circulation

1. Implement regular physical activity of skeletal muscles especially of the lower extremities to facilitate the movement of venous blood. For example, active and passive exercises of the legs improve venous return and minimize the complications associated with venous stasis. Physical activity increases the physical fitness of the heart and skeletal muscles to more efficiently move the blood through the vascular system. New vessels are gradually formed to circumvent a localized narrowing (collateral circulation fig. 3-9).

2. Eliminate cigarette smoking to prevent vasoconstriction and reduce one of the risk factors associated with the development of cardiovascular and pulmonary disease.

3. Control hyperlipidemia and cholesterol levels to prevent the progression of atherosclerosis.

4. Avoid cold environmental temperatures. Provide for warmth without applying external heat. As peripheral neural receptors may be impaired, there is increased risk for tissue injury from heating pads and hot baths.

5. Teach the individual to assess their fingers and toes daily for circulatory adequacy: peripheral pulses, edema, skin temperature, and capillary refill.

6. Teach good hygienic care of the feet to prevent any skin breakdown. Wear comfortable fitting shoes to prevent blisters. Keep the feet clean and dry, using mild soap and warm water. Apply mild lotion to prevent dryness. Keep the feet warm with clean, loose-fitting socks. Corns, calluses and toenails should be cared for cautiously to minimize injury.

7. A break in the skin should be reported to the physician for prompt treatment. Impaired neural receptors may mask serious tissue injury. Delayed healing is often associated with impaired peripheral circulation.

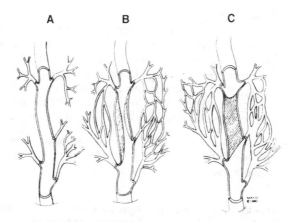

*Fig. 3-9. **Vessel occlusion with collateral circulation:** (A) Open, functioning artery; (B) Partial artery closure with collateral circulation being established; (C) Total artery occlusion with collateral circulation bypassing the occlusion. From S.M. Lewis, I.C. Collier: <u>Medical-Surgical Nursing: Assessment and Mangement of Clinical Problems</u>, 4th ed.; St. Louis: Mosby-Year Book, Inc., 1995. Reprinted with permission. Courtesy Mayo Clinic, Rochester, Minn.*

Common Clinical Examples

1. Arterial insufficiency

    — Atherosclerotic placque formation with resultant tissue hypoxia distal to the occlusion is the most common cause of arterial insufficiency. The most common sites are the common iliac artery just below the bifurcation of the abdominal aorta, femoral artery and the popliteal artery. Localized lesions can be identified by angiography and surgical by-pass grafts may be performed to restore distal circulation.

    — Impaired circulation may lead to skin breakdown (ulcer formation) or gangrene. A pregangrenous extremity appears pale and feels cold. These symptoms are unaffected by position or pressure changes. A necrotic, gangrenous extremity or portion of an extremity appears black, shriveled and hard.

    — An extremity may become potentially gangrenous without the individual being aware of the situation when the arterial insufficiency has developed gradually. Progressive loss of neural pain receptors mask the severity of the circulatory impairment. A minor tissue injury and associated delayed healing may quickly progress to extensive tissue damage and the necessity for amputation.

2. Varicose veins
   - Structural weakness of the walls or valves within the veins lead to stretched or dilated vessels. The valves no longer promote the forward flow of venous blood toward the heart, and retrograde flow and back pressure causes further dilation. Ultimately the veins become enlarged and tortuous. Varicosities are most common in the saphenous veins of the legs but may also occur in the esophageal and hemorrhoidal veins.

   - Predisposing factors include: family history, advanced age, prolonged sitting or standing, obesity, pregnancy, constricting garments, and conditions causing increased intra-abdominal pressure (large tumors, ascites).

   - Due to the impaired venous return, there is an increased risk for thrombosis formation and subsequent embolization traveling and lodging in the lungs.

   - Measures to decrease the risk for development are the most effective preventive interventions. The injection of sclerosing agents leads to the occlusion of a localized varicosed vein. Surgical ligation and stripping of the affected vein is another intervention for more extensive vessel involvement. Effective preventive measures usually minimize the recurrence.

   - Instructions for applying anti-embolic stockings should include:
     - Apply stockings when the veins are most likely to be empty; e.g. after the individual has been recumbent or legs elevated for 20 minutes to minimize distention.
     - Ensure that the tops of the stockings do not roll as this will act as a tourniquet and further impair circulation.
     - Avoid wrinkles and creases in the stockings.
     - Avoid acute flexion of joints and a prolonged sitting position. Avoid crossed legs.

3. Phlebitis (inflammation of a vein)
   - Although venous thrombosis and thrombophlebitis are different disorders, clinically they are referred to interchangeably. Sometimes the inflammation (phlebitis) occurs first, which leads to the development of a blood clot. Other times the thrombosis develops first, which causes the inflammation of the affected vein.

   - Inflammation of a superficial vein is a frequent complication of intravenous (IV) therapy especially when the cannula remains in one location beyond 72 hours. Veins in the hands are less likely to become inflamed than veins in the feet. IV fluids with antibiotics and potassium chloride are associated with an increased incidence of phlebitis.

— Phlebitis of deep veins is secondary to a thrombosis or blood clot and place the individual at risk for emboli formation which may travel to the lungs (pulmonary emboli).

— Risk factors associated with deep vein thrombosis (DVT) include:

- Presence of varicose veins.

- Increased age.

- Inactivity especially following extensive surgical procedures such as orthopedic surgery and trauma.

- Serious infections and some malignancies due to increased coagulability.

- Injury or manipulation of the vessels, especially during some gynecological surgical procedures.

- Estrogen therapy and oral contraceptives.

- Cigarette smoking.

— Measures to prevent the occurrence of DVT include: early ambulation and leg exercises; anti-embolic stockings and low-dose anticoagulant therapy for high risk individuals.

- 5000 units of subcutaneous heparin is administered 2-3 times per day during prolonged bedrest of high-risk individuals. Partial thromboplastin times (PTT) are obtained to ensure prophylactic coagulation levels.

- Aspirin may be prescribed for its anti-aggregation action on platelets.

- Dextran IV solution may be administered as a prophylactic anticoagulant for persons for whom bleeding would be detrimental such as in neurosurgical clinical situations.

— Treatment measures are directed toward preventing further clot formation:

- Subcutaneous or intravenous heparin with dosages titrated by serial partial thromboplastin times (PTT) to achieve 2-3 times the normal range to prevent the extension or buildup of the existing clot.

- Occasionally, thrombolytic agents such as streptokinase or urokinase may be used to dissolve an established clot that is occluding a major vessel.

- Surgical removal (thrombectomy) is seldom necessary.

- A transvenous device may be surgically placed in the vena cava to catch emboli before they reach the heart. The umbrella-like device is indicated for individuals with recurrent DVT and a history of pulmonary emboli.

— If an individual is discharged on anticoagulant (Coumadin) therapy, instructions should include:

- Clearly stated information about the name of the anticoagulant, its purpose, dosage and schedule of administration, precautions and potential side effects.

- Take medication as prescribed without changing the dosage or skipping a day unless directed by the physician.

- Maintain the schedule for laboratory tests; prothrombin time (PT).

- Wear a Medi-Alert bracelet.

- Avoid alcohol consumption or dietary changes which may alter the response to the anticoagulant.

- Avoid taking over-the-counter medications that contain aspirin without consulting the physician. Anticoagulant effect may be potentiated.

- Report the occurrence of any of the following symptoms: hematuria, melena, epistaxis, ecchymosis.

- Inform other physicians and dentists of the anticoagulant therapy when making appointments and seeking treatment of other conditions.

4. Secondary skin breakdown

— Stasis ulcers are due to poor venous return, congestion of deoxygenated blood and buildup of end products of cellular metabolism. This complication is secondary to severe varicose veins or recurrent thrombophlebitis.

- The skin appears darkly pigmented with local edema. The texture becomes leathery with localized pain when the extremity is dependent. Skin breakdown usually occurs in the area of the ankle.

— Peripheral arterial insufficiency or occlusion leads to varying degrees of impaired perfusion and delivery of oxygen and cellular nutrients. The tissue distal to the occluded site becomes ischemic and eventually necrotic (gangrene). This complication is secondary to atherosclerosis or advanced diabetes mellitus.

- The skin appears pale or blanched and the skin surface becomes shiny and taut with progressive loss of hair. The peripheral pulses are diminished or absent. Ischemic skin breakdown usually begins with the toes.

- Vascular by-pass grafts may be performed to improve localized arterial circulation (femoral-popliteal by-pass or femoral-posterior tibial by-pass).

SECTION 5: HEMATOLOGICAL DYSFUNCTION

Overview of Disrupted Blood Component Function

Erythrocyte dysfunction is a result of too many RBCs (polycythemia), too few RBCs (anemia), or cell structure defects (sickle-cell syndrome). When there is an excess of RBCs in circulation, the blood has thicker viscosity. Consequently, the movement or circulation is slowed increasing the risk for clot formation (thrombosis). The subsequent occlusion may occur in an artery or a vein.

When there are insufficient numbers or ineffective RBCs in circulation, the amount of circulating hemoglobin is inadequate. Sometimes a shortened RBC life cycle or increased cell destruction (hemolytic anemia) is the cause. Too few RBCs or too little hemoglobin produce symptoms of tissue hypoxia and altered cellular metabolism. With a sudden loss of blood components such as with hemorrhage, symptoms of tissue hypoxia are dramatic. Immediate volume replacement is needed (saline solutions, plasma or volume expanders). Transfusion of fresh whole blood is preferred as it contains clotting factors.

Leukocytes are the primary internal defenders against infection and other foreign invasion. Normally, there is an increase in WBCs in circulation when a microorganism invades the body. When this response does not occur, relatively minor invaders proliferate and serious opportunistic infections develop. Too few (leukopenia) or ineffective WBCs increase the risk of this complication. An excess of WBCs (leukocytosis) as seen in some forms of leukemia cause other circulatory problems. Increased numbers of WBCs increase the blood viscosity, white clots may form and vessel occlusion may occur.

Inadequate numbers of platelets in circulation is called thrombocytopenia. With low numbers, there is an increased risk for spontaneous bleeding. Bruises (ecchymoses) or small areas of bleeding in the skin (petechiae) are observable with low platelet counts. Similar bleeding may also be occurring internally in gastrointestinal or respiratory tracts or from capillaries in the brain.

Assessment of Suspected Hematological Dysfunction

1. History of symptoms and chemical/drug exposure

   — Many prescribed and over-the-counter medications are known to produce hematologic effects and bone marrow suppression. Periodic use of analgesics, tranquilizers, laxatives and sedatives are overlooked by persons when asked about the medications that they are taking.

   — As a fever is a common manifestation of many hematologic disorders, identification of a pattern of occurrence is helpful. For example, night time sweating may be associated with a fever which is a characteristic pattern of Hodgkin's disease.

2. General appearance

   — As many hematological disorders cause a decrease in RBCs, there is progressive fatigue and malaise. The severity of clinical fatigability is more related to the rate of onset rather than the degree of RBC or Hgb loss. For example, some individuals are able to carry on their activities of daily living in spite of a progressive decrease in Hgb levels to less than 8 G/dl. Whereas, other individuals may exhibit severe fatigue and exertional dyspnea with a sudden drop of 2 G/dl in Hgb value to 12 G/dl.

   — Due to decreased or altered function of WBCs, there is a progressive lowered resistance to infections and increased time for healing. Relatively minor infections, such as a common cold or urinary tract infections, linger and/or recur.

   — Due to decreased or altered function of platelets, there is an increase in bruising from relatively minor injuries. Spontaneous nosebleeds or prolonged menses may occur.

3. Changes in the skin

   — Petechiae, ecchymoses and purpura are associated with decreased platelet counts (thrombocytopenia).

   — Jaundice may be observed in the sclera, conjunctiva and oral mucosa. It is suggestive of rapid destruction of RBCs and pernicious anemia.

   — With iron-deficiency anemia, the individual will notice dry skin, dry hair and brittle nails.

- Severe itching (pruritus) is associated with Hodgkin's disease and polycythemia vera.

4. Head and neck

   - When jaundice of the sclera or pallor of the conjunctiva are observed, the individual often will have visual disturbances.

   - A smooth or sensitive surface of the tongue is associated with pernicious anemia and nutritional deficiencies.

   - The neck should be assessed closely for the presence of lymph node enlargement and tenderness. Lymph node enlargement often is the reason for seeking medical attention.

5. Chest

   - Lung fields and heart sounds are WNL.

   - Tenderness of the sternum may be identified with individuals with the leukemic processes.

6. Abdomen

   - Enlarged liver and/or spleen may be noted.

7. Extremities

   - Bone and joint pain may be noted.

Diagnostic Studies

1. Extensive blood work to identify all blood components and their microscopic features is performed. RBCs are described by cell size (macrocytic, normocytic, microcytic) and by hemoglobin concentration (normochromic or hypochromic).

2. Bone marrow aspiration or biopsy is a sterile procedure to determine cell analysis. The common sites are the sternum, iliac crest and tibia.

Measures to Restore Hematological Function

1. Medication

   - Iron replacement (ferrous sulfate or ferrous gluconate) usually restores 2/3 of the hemoglobin deficit within 4-6 weeks.

   - Inferon injections must be administered by Z track to decrease irritation to subcutaneous tissue.

   - Elevated reticulocyte count is a good indicator or response to iron therapy.

2. Blood transfusion therapy

    Blood transfusion has become a major public concern in recent years. Homologous transfusion is the standard transfusion from random volunteer donors. Autologous transfusion is the use of the individual's own blood either by donation just prior to a time needed or by salvaging RBCs with "cell saver" devices. Blood components may be separated and administered for specific uses.

    — Specific policies and procedures must be followed regarding the administration of blood and blood products. Some procedures are specific to an institution. General considerations include:

    • Verification of the correct blood product with person/recipient is a nursing responsibility. Accurate administration and assessment of the person's response are also nursing responsibilities.

    • Normal saline (0.9%) is the only crystalloid solution that can be administered with blood and components. All medications are incompatible with blood products and cause agglutination and/or hemolysis of RBCs.

    • Start the infusion rate slowly (2 ml/minute) for the first 15-30 minutes and obtain vital signs. Most adverse reactions occur during the initial administration.

3. Bone marrow transplantation

    This is an accepted treatment for aplastic or sickle-cell anemias and many malignant disorders. The donation is cell typed and matched to the recipient. A relative especially a twin usually has the closest cell compatibility for successful donation. There is less incidence of rejection complications as compared to other tissue/organ transplantation procedures.

Common Clinical Examples

1. Anemias

    — This is a common hematopoietic disorder involving a reduced number of RBCs or reduced amount of hemoglobin. The general effects result from a reduced oxygen-carrying capacity and subsequent tissue hypoxia. Fatigue and dyspnea are the most common clinical manifestations.

    — Iron-deficiency anemia is the most common anemia and is commonly associated with inadequate dietary intake or blood loss from malignancies and prolonged menses. Small amounts of on-going loss, especially from the gastrointestinal tract, may go undetected until significant anemia is present.

- Iron replacement or blood transfusion are common therapies.

— Pernicious anemia is due to inadequate supply or utilization of Vitamin B_{12} or a decrease in the production of intrinsic factor by the gastric mucosa. As neural tissue is particularly sensitive to B_{12} deficiency, paresthesia and subtle ataxia are common. This is a megaloblastic anemia in which the RBCs are large and immature.

- Schillings's test is specific for this anemia. Radioactive Vitamin B_{12} is administered. With pernicious anemia, the B_{12} is not absorbed and the urine levels are low.

- Vitamin B_{12} (cyanocobalamin) replacement is the treatment of choice and may need to be administered regularly for long periods of time to ensure an adequate blood count.

— Sickle-cell anemia is a genetic disorder of abnormal Hgb which causes RBCs to become crescent shaped. In response to episodes of tissue hypoxia, the abnormally shaped cells aggregated and occlude vessels in the microcirculation which precipitates further episodes of tissue hypoxia. Most sickled erythrocytes regain a normal shape after reoxygenation and hydration.

- Hemolytic crisis occurs when a large number of RBCs are destroyed. Acute physiological and psychological stress precipitate a crisis. Clinical manifestations include: jaundice, dyspnea, joint or abdominal pain, decreasing blood pressure and increasing heart rate.

- Steroids are often prescribed to decrease the occurrence of crisis episodes.

— Aplastic (hypoplastic) anemia results from an inability of the bone marrow to produce sufficient numbers of RBCs. Approximately half of the individuals with this type of anemia acquired it secondary to antineoplastic or antimicrobial (e.g. Chloramphenicol) therapy or radiation therapy. The remaining individuals have a concurrent immunological disorder.

- Most individuals have pancytopenia, depression of all bone marrow elements: erythrocytes, platelets, granulocytes and neutrophils. Bleeding tendencies and susceptibility to infections are common indicators.

2. Polycythemia
   - This chronic disorder is characterized by excessive production of red blood cells. As the number of RBCs increases, the blood volume, blood viscosity and hemoglobin concentration increases. There is an associated high risk for thrombosis formation.

   - Polycythemia vera is a primary disorder of unknown etiology. Secondary polycythemia is a physiological response to chronic hypoxia. This is a physiological compensation attempt to increase the circulation of oxygen.

   - Clinical manifestations are associated with intravascular overload and congestive heart failure. For example, hypertension, headache, dizziness, visual disturbances and chest pain are common. Nocturnal dyspnea, crackles, and chest pain are related to the impaired left ventricular function. Ruddy (reddened) complexion and hepatosplenomegaly are associated with venous congestion. Thrombophlebitis and joint pain are associated with the increased blood viscosity and coagulability.

   - Phlebotomy to reduce the blood volume and lower the hematocrit (Hct) to 45% often results in marked improvement of clinical symptoms. Myelosuppressive agents (radiophosphorus) are administered to inhibit the proliferation of RBCs. Alkalating agents (busulfan and chlorambucil) are administered to decrease bone marrow function.

3. Neoplastic disorders of the hematopoietic system
   The major types of neoplastic disorders are presented in this unit and the care of adults with oncological conditions is discussed in Unit 8. The chemotherapeutic agents and treatment modalities are also discussed in Unit 8.

   - Hodgkin's disease is a malignant condition involving lymph tissue and is distinguished from other lymphomas by the presence of Reed-Sternberg cells. It affects young adults and is characterized by an insidious onset of non-specific symptoms.

     • With early diagnosis and chemotherapeutic treatment, a long-term survival (20 years) is now possible.

     • Staging is done to determine the extent of involvement. Lymph node involvement on the same side of the diaphragm is associated with more favorable prognosis.

   - Acute leukemia is an abnormal, malignant proliferation of WBCs which accumulate in the bone marrow, body tissues and blood vessels and eventually impair the functioning of other blood components. The type of leukemia is categorized by cell type.

- Acute myelocytic leukemia (AML) usually affects adults older than 20 years of age. The goal of chemotherapy is to produce a remission or reduction of malignant cells and restoration of normal hematopoiesis.

  – Chronic leukemia occurs later in adult life and progresses more slowly. This type is also categorized by cell type. Although affected persons survive longer and the severity of symptoms is less, the same principles of care and management apply.

4. Coagulation disorders

   At the time of a vascular injury, platelets adhere to each other to form a temporary plug to stop local bleeding. In addition, platelets play a major role in the sequence of reactions in clot formation.

   – Thrombocytopenia is a decrease in the number of platelets in circulation. It may occur as a result of decreased production, increased loss or increased use during increased coagulation.

     - Triggering situations include: autoimmune disorder, severe vascular injury, spleen malfunction, side effects of certain chemotherapeutic agents or antibiotics.

     - A platelet count below 100,000 is significant and is associated with increased skin injury and bruises. With a count below 20,000, there is a serious risk for spontaneous hemorrhage.

     - Avoid venipuncture and IM injections when possible. Pressure for 5-10 minutes at injection site is usually required to stop bleeding.

     - Platelet concentration, cryoprecipitate or fresh frozen plasma may be administered to replace platelets or clotting factors.

   – DIC (Disseminated Intravascular Coagulation) is an acute coagulation disorder characterized by increased clotting in the microcirculation and hemorrhage. It is a secondary disorder or a complication of another pathology which usually involves massive clot formation. Available platelets are used in the formation of multiple systemic clots. While most high-risk clinical situations are cared for in critical care settings, occasionally it may occur with general medical-surgical clinical situations.

- High-risk clinical situations include individuals with: major infections (sepsis), liver disease (cirrhosis, hepatic necrosis), major surgery, trauma, massive transfusion therapy, immune suppression, pulmonary emboli, neoplasms, or hemorrhagic pancreatitis.

- Clinical manifestations include: abrupt onset of bleeding, oozing from venipuncture sites or mucosa, hematuria, unusual bruising to minor injury.

unit *4*

NURSING CARE OF ADULTS WITH

Digestive Conditions

T*his unit addresses a wide range of common, recurring conditions of adults which affect the functioning of the gastrointestinal system. The care of individuals with some degree of
impaired digestive dysfunction on general medical-surgical nursing
units is addressed. The management and care of critical and
unstable conditions which require continuous monitoring and multiple intravenous infusions are usually cared for in specialty care
units and are not addressed in this unit. Examples of clinical
conditions requiring high acuity care include necrotic bowel syndrome and perforated bowel.*

SECTION 1: OVERVIEW

Effective plans for care are based upon an understanding of the normal functioning of the digestive system. The alimentary canal or gastrointestinal tract is a long tube that connects the mouth to the anus. The digestive system also includes accessory organs: liver, gallbladder and the exocrine component of the pancreas. The functional categories related to this system include ingestion (taking in food and liquids), digestion (food breakdown), absorption (transport of nutrients into the circulatory system), and elimination (removal of food residue).

Psychological and emotional factors may impair digestive functioning and produce characteristic symptoms such as anorexia, indigestion, diarrhea or constipation. Eating habits and sharing food with friends are integral to social interactions. Physiological changes which alter eating and elimination activities impact on an individual's interaction with others. Therefore, the psychosocial component of gastrointestinal tract dysfunction cannot be overlooked and may be a cause of noncompliance.

Anatomical Considerations of the Digestive System

1. Oral component
    — An adequate number of functioning teeth and the presence of healthy gums are essential for the intake of food. Sufficient chewing action prepares food into particles for digestion. Coordinated neurological activity is required for swallowing without causing a choking response or aspiration into the trachea and respiratory tract.

    — Three pairs of salivary glands secrete about 1 liter (1000 ml) of saliva every day. Saliva is comprised mostly of water and varying amounts of mucus, some electrolytes and a carbohydrate-digesting enzyme (ptyalin).

2. Esophagus
    — This hollow muscular tube connects the oropharynx with the stomach. It passes through the thorax and diaphragm. The entrance to the stomach is governed by a constricting muscle (cardiac sphincter) which controls the passage of swallowed food. Due to greater pressures within the stomach, this muscle normally prevents regurgitation of gastric contents back into the esophagus.

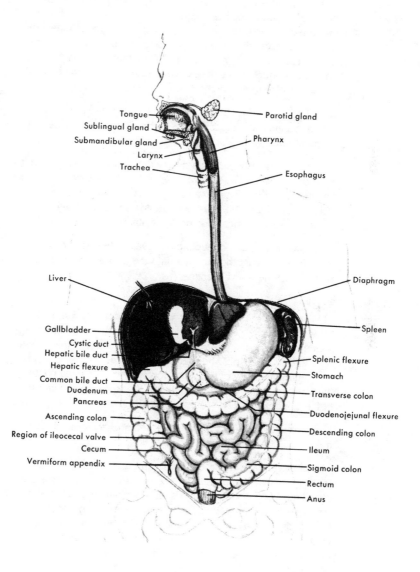

Fig. 4-1. Organs of the GI System. From C. Anthony, G. Thibodeau: *Textbook of Anatomy and Physiology;* St. Louis: Mosby-Year Book, Inc., 1987. Reprinted with permission.

3. Stomach
   — This hollow, muscular structure stores food particles after swallowing. Its size can increase to accommodate various volumes of ingested food and liquids. The stomach is located in
   the upper left quadrant of the abdomen. It secretes digestive
   enzymes, mixes the food particles and moves the partially digested food (chyme) into the small intestine. The pyloric
   sphincter controls the exit of chyme from the stomach into the
   small intestine (duodenum).

   — About 1500-3000 ml of gastric juice are secreted each day. At
   rest or during a nondigestive state, the stomach contains only
   50 ml of fluid.

   — The wall of the stomach has a very rich blood supply with an
   abundant collateral vascular system. The fundus or upper portion contains the primary secretory units. Interrelated neural
   sequences trigger the release of gastric secretion of hydrochlo-
   ric acid, pepsin, intrinsic factor and histamine.

   — The pyloric sphincter controls the movement of gastric contents (chyme) from the stomach into the duodenum or the first
   segment of the small intestine.

4. Small intestine
   — This segment of the tube system is approximately 5 meters or
   22 feet in length. It is functionally divided into the duodenum,
   jejunum and ileum. The small intestine begins with the duodenum in the upper mid-abdomen. The ileocecal valve or sphincter controls the flow of intestinal contents from the ileum into
   the large intestine which is located in the lower right quadrant
   of the abdomen.

   — Approximately 3000 ml of intestinal secretions are produced
   daily.

   — The peritoneum is a serous membrane that surrounds and protects the abdominal organs as the pericardium and pleura surround the heart and lungs. The visceral peritoneum lies over
   the organs and the parietal peritoneum lines the outer wall of
   the abdominal cavity. Inflammation of the peritoneum is called
   peritonitis. Healing may lead to ring-like scar formations between the peritoneum and underlying organs which are called
   adhesions.

5. Large intestine
   — This last segment of the tubing system is approximately 1.5
   meters or 5-6 feet in length. The cecum is a pouch that receives the chyme from the ileum. The appendix is a small ap-
   pendage attached to the cecum. The colon consists of four

parts: the ascending colon, the transverse colon and the descending colon. The remaining segments include the sigmoid, rectum and anus. External and internal rings of sphincter muscles comprise the anus.

6. Liver

   — This is one of the largest organs in the body and is located under the right side of the diaphragm. Its metabolic functions require large quantities of blood; therefore, approximately 400-500 ml of oxygenated blood is delivered to the liver every minute (about 15% of the cardiac output). The hepatic portal vein receives deoxygenated blood from the venous system at a rate of 1000-1200 ml per minute.

   — The liver assists intestinal digestion by secreting 700-1200 ml of bile per day. The majority of bile is stored in the gallbladder and is released as needed for fat digestion. One component of bile is bilirubin which is an end product of red blood cell break-down.

   — The liver acts as a large warehouse of reserve supplies. It stores certain vitamins (A, D, E, K and B$_{12}$). Iron is stored as ferritin. Energy sources from glucose metabolism are stored as glycogen.

   — The liver has the capacity to reproduce its cellular structures or has regenerative capability. However, with repeated cellular damage, fibrous tissue replacement may occur. Depending upon the degree of fibrous replacement, hepatic function may eventually be impaired (cirrhosis of the liver).

7. Gallbladder

   — This sac-like structure is located between the liver and the duodenum. The primary purposes are storing and concentrating bile until it is needed for fat digestion. It holds about 30-90 ml of bile. A duct system connects the liver and gallbladder with the duodenum at the Ampulla of Vater.

8. Exocrine pancreas

   — The pancreas is composed of two major anatomical and physiological functional units. The exocrine component includes the cells and ducts to secrete and deliver enzymes and alkaline fluids to the duodenum for digestive purposes.

   — The pancreas is approximately 20 cm in length and lies deep in the abdomen. Its head lies within the curve of the duodenum and its tail lies behind the stomach and extends to the spleen in the upper left quadrant.

— The bicarbonate (HCO_3-) concentration of the pancreatic secretions varies between 50-120 mEq/Liter. This highly alkalotic juice neutralizes the acidic chyme as it leaves the stomach and activates intestinal and pancreatic enzymes.

— Approximately 700 ml of pancreatic secretions are produced every day.

Normal Physiological Functioning of the Digestive System

1. Food breakdown begins in the mouth with the mixing of small food particles with saliva. The taste buds on the tongue and olfactory nerves in the nose are continuously stimulated which add to the satisfaction of eating.

2. Stomach

   — The rate of movement or peristalsis is approximately three waves per minute. This motility depends upon the volume, osmotic pressure and chemical composition of the contents. The greater the caloric density of the ingested food, the more slowly the stomach empties.

   — The pH of gastric contents is very acidic; usually 3.0- 5.0. This degree of acidity is required for pepsin activity and the digestion of proteins. This acidity also inhibits bacterial growth; therefore the stomach is relatively sterile.

3. Small intestine

   — The inside surface of the small intestine is covered with tiny mucosal folds or villi which are the functional units for absorption. Digestive enzymes are secreted and nutrients are absorbed. The pH of intestinal contents is very alkaline with a pH range of 7.0-9.0.

   — The mucosal surface of the small intestine is normally replaced every 4-7 days. This rapid cellular replacement makes the intestinal mucosa very sensitive to radiation and chemotherapy, which disrupt cell division.

   — Digestion continues in the proximal or first segment of the small intestine (duodenum). The presence of bile salts, pancreatic enzymes and intestinal enzymes enhance the process.

   — The body's daily requirements for vitamins and minerals are obtained from dietary intake. They are absorbed from the small intestine. The fat soluble vitamins (A, D, E and K) require the presence of bile salts for adequate absorption.

Most water-soluble vitamins (B complex, C and folic acid) are readily absorbed. Vitamin B_{12} (cyanocobalamin) also requires the presence of the intrinsic factor which is secreted from the wall of the stomach for adequate absorption to occur.

— Digested nutrients (glucose, amino acids and fatty acids) along with water, vitamins and electrolytes cross the intestinal mucosa and move into the villi capillaries. Most substances are first transported to the liver for detoxification or storage. The remaining intestinal contents continue to move along the tubing system toward the large intestine by peristaltic activity.

— Chyme usually moves through the small intestine in 3-10 hours. However, a "peristaltic rush" may occur in which a powerful wave moves contents from the duodenum to the ileocecal valve within a few minutes. This is a physiological response to remove potentially harmful substances through the system with minimal time for digestion or absorption to occur.

4. Large intestine
   — Approximately 500-700 ml of chyme arrives at the cecum each day. Slow transport through the large intestine allows for efficient water and electrolyte absorption.

   — Most of the water is absorbed as large intestinal contents moves toward the rectum. A semi-solid mass of food residue, unabsorbed secretions, epithelial cells and bacteria remains. The presence of this fecal mass in the sigmoid colon stimulates the defecation reflex.

     • Voluntary suppression of defecation is achieved by contracting the muscles of the pelvic floor and external anal sphincter. Elimination can be augmented by increasing intra-abdominal pressure and forced holding on expiration (Valsalva maneuver). Bradycardia and increased intracranial pressure (IICP) may accompany this straining activity.

   — There are increasing types and numbers of bacteria along the intestinal tract. This normal flora or growth of bacteria such as *Escherichia coli* and *Streptococcus* participate in the metabolism of carbohydrates and lipids. The number of normal bacteria is highest in the large intestine.

   — Decreased peristalsis can lead to an overpopulation of bacteria and malabsorption of vitamins and nutrients. Damage or injury to the intestinal wall may lead to leakage of intestinal contents and bacteria into surrounding tissue which can be very irritating or infectious.

5. Liver
   - This anatomical structure is very active in many physiological processes. Because it normally contains large volumes of blood for its metabolic functions, it also can control the storage or release of vascular volumes in the event of a circulatory deficit (shock or hemorrhage).

   - Plasma proteins (albumin, globulin) are synthesized or made in the liver. These proteins normally circulate throughout the vascular compartment providing a fluid holding function. They maintain intravascular fluid volume and blood pressure.

   - Kupffer cells in the liver act as master filters to remove bacteria and foreign particles from the portal (venous) blood.

   - Clotting factors (prothrombin, fibrinogen) are synthesized and stored in the liver. Vitamin K acts in the liver as a catalyst to promote prothrombin synthesis, which is necessary for effective clotting.

   - The liver also alters the toxicity of many substances that may be present in the body. This metabolic detoxification process also prevents the accumulation and adverse effects of potentially harmful substances and facilitates intestinal and renal excretion without causing damage to these structures.

6. Gallbladder
   - This structure is a storehouse for bile. It contracts and releases bile in response to the presence of fatty foods in the stomach and small intestine.

   - The majority of bile salts that move through the small intestine are absorbed from the ileum and transported back to the liver for reuse.

7. Exocrine pancreas
   - The release of pancreatic enzymes into the duodenum is triggered by presence of food in the stomach and intestine. Trypsin is a protein-digesting enzyme. Amylase is a carbohydrate-digesting enzyme. Lipase is a fat-reducing or emulsifying enzyme. These enzymes are effective in alkaline solutions of a 7.0-9.0 pH range.

Variations Related to Aging

1. Age-related changes in gastrointestinal function may begin by age 50. Teeth are lost primarily due to preventable periodontal (gum) disease. As the number of taste buds decline and the sense of smell diminishes, eating becomes less pleasurable.

- Anorexia and altered nutritional status may lead to nutritional anemia, obesity, vitamin and/or mineral deficiencies.

2. Gastric motility and acid content of gastric juices declines. Smaller and more frequent food intake is better tolerated by elders. Food substances are digested and nutrients are absorbed more slowly.

3. Although constipation is a frequent complaint, it is probably due to decreased intake of fluids and dietary roughage rather than physiological factors. Changes in dietary habits and increased physical activity are effective preventive measures.

4. Liver and pancreatic function remain within normal parameters as age progresses. However, the metabolism of drugs is slowed which may result in higher drug levels in circulation, causing varying degrees of toxicity.

    - Pancreatic enzyme secretion becomes slowed after age 40 with a decrease in lipase activity. The composition of bile becomes more prone to stone formation with age. Therefore, intolerance to dietary fat intake increases.

5. Several factors are related to progressive bone loss among elders. Dietary intake of calcium often decreases. Also decreasing levels of circulating Vitamin D are common. This vitamin is needed for the intestinal absorption of calcium.

6. Malabsorption may occur among the elderly which is thought to be associated with the bacterial colonization in the duodenum which interfers with absorption. Clinically these changes may predispose elders to impaired wound healing following injury, surgery or trauma.

SECTION 2: DIGESTIVE DYSFUNCTION

Overview

Alterations in the functioning of the gastrointestinal tract are related to disruption or cessation of physiological activity of the segment of the tract involved. Normal anatomy and physiology provides the basis for comparison of symptoms and assessment findings. Therefore if the health care provider understands normal findings, the presence of other findings suggests physiological dysfunction and possible pathology.

Assessment of Gastrointestinal (GI) Status

1. Nutritional information

   — Dietary recall or a diary of intake reveals the quantity and quality of nutrients ingested during a 24-hour period. Recommended dietary allowances serve as guidelines for minimum daily intake of selected nutrients according to age.

2. General information

   — Obtaining a history of symptoms, self-care measures and over-the-counter self medication is essential. Many gastrointestinal symptoms are self treated for some time before medical assistance is sought. Usually persistent pain, diarrhea, constipation or the presence of blood triggers seeking medical advise.

   — Patterns of unexplained symptoms such as indigestion, anorexia, belching (eructation), "bloating" (distention), passing flatulence and bowel elimination irregularity provide clues to changes in physiological functioning.

   — Patterns in weight gain or weight loss without changes in dietary intake are pertinent. The use of height/weight tables, body weight indices, skinfold thickness and wrist measurements provide guidelines for ideal body weight according to body frame or bone structure.

3. Presence of symptoms of altered GI function

   — Pain is a frequent symptom of GI dysfunction. The character, duration, frequency, and time of occurrence vary greatly. Associated factors and alleviating measures need to be identified.

   — Indigestion is one type of pain that may be associated with eating or not eating. It originates in the upper quadrants of the abdomen usually below the sternum. Eating fatty foods often is the cause as caloric dense foods remain in the stomach longer than carbohydrates or proteins. Coarse vegetables or spicy foods may contribute to this symptom.

     • Many over-the-counter preparations are available for self treatment. Frequent and repeated use may mask the symptoms of a more serious condition.

   — Intestinal "gas" (belching or flatulence) may be attributed to the intake of certain foods, altered digestion or decreased peristaltic activity. Excess "gas" may contribute to a distended abdomen or "bloated" feeling.

     • When belching is accompanied by gastric juices, a burning sensation ("heartburn") may be detected by the individual.

- Vomiting (reverse peristalsis) is a physiological response to remove potentially harmful substances from the GI tract. It usually is preceded by nausea.

    • When the vomited contents (emesis) contains blood, it is called hematemesis. If the blood has mixed with gastric contents, the appearance of emesis is brownish liquid or contains brownish flecks giving the emesis the appearance of "coffee grounds".

- Diarrhea refers to the abnormal increase in the frequency and consistency of bowel elimination. When movement through the large intestine is faster than normal, less than normal amounts of water and electrolytes are absorbed. The bowel contents arrive at the rectum in a liquid state.

    • When undigested fat progresses through the GI tract, it causes a characteristic type of diarrhea (steatorrhea). This abnormal stool composition is due to insufficient pancreatic enzyme activity.

    • When blood progresses through the GI tract, it changes the color and composition of the stool. Black, tarry stool is indicative of bleeding higher in the tract. Small amounts of blood in the stool can be detected by simple, non-invasive, bedside analysis of a stool sample (stool for occult blood).

    • When bile does not reach the small intestine, the color of the stool changes to a pale, clay color without a change in consistency.

4. As the majority of the GI tract is located within the abdominal cavity, a systematic assessment of this region of the body is required.

    - The abdominal skin surface should be smooth without the presence of distended blood vessels, jaundice or petechiae (small capillary hemorrhages which do not blanch with pressure). The abdomen feels soft.

    - Bowel sounds should be noted every 5 to 15 seconds and should be heard (auscultated) in all quadrants. The presence of vascular sounds such as bruits may suggest a serious major vessel problem. The abdomen should be auscultated then palpated to avoid stimulation of bowel sounds.

    - Systemic organs such as the liver, gallbladder or spleen are not usually palpated. If the edge of the liver is felt below the right rib cage, it is measured in finger widths. For example, 1+ would refer to one finger width below the lower right rib.

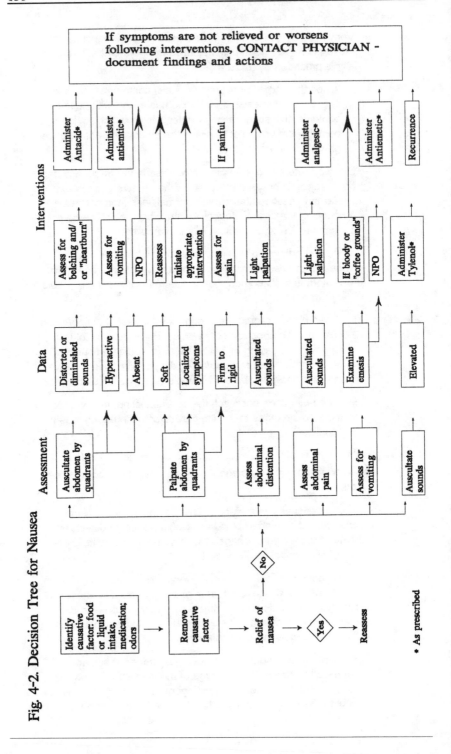

Fig 4-2. Decision Tree for Nausea

- The inguinal area or fold between the abdomen and thigh
  should be inspected and palpated for possible protrusions.
  The internal anatomical openings in this area for major vessels
  create the potential for a loop of intestine to protrude (inguinal
  or femoral hernia).

- The external orifice of the anus is inspected for any discoloriza-
  tion, lesions, hemorrhoids or prolapse of rectal tissue. A digital examination may be warranted if fecal impaction is
  suspected.

Diagnostic Testing of GI Status

1. Visualization procedures
   - With the use of fiberoptic tubing, the upper or lower segments
     of the tract may be directly observed (endoscopy or col-
     onoscopy). An esophagogastroduodenoscopy (EGD) involves
     the direct viewing of the esophagus, stomach and first seg-
     ment of the small intestine. A colonoscopy refers to the direct
     viewing of the large intestine. A proctoscopy and sigmoidos-
     copy involves the direct viewing of the distal segments of the
     large intestine.

   - Radiographic visualization by filling segments of the tract with
     contrast liquid and taking serial x-rays reveals anatomical con-
     tours. A barium enema is a lower GI series, whereas a bar-
     ium swallow is an upper GI series. A cholecystogram
     visualizes the gallbladder; whereas a cholangiogram visualizes
     the bile duct system.

   - Abdominal organs may also be scanned by non-invasive tech-
     niques such as ultrasound or computerized tomography proce-
     dures (CAT scans or MRI).

2. Various laboratory tests may be conducted to determine organ
   function. For example, the liver has many physiological functions
   that are reflected in blood testing. For example, changes in the
   prothrombin time, albumin levels, bilirubin levels or enzymes may
   indicate liver dysfunction.

3. Exocrine function of the pancreas is assessed by determining
   selected enzyme activity. For example, amylase and lipasl levels
   in the serum and intestinal secretions are obtained and measured.

Measures to Improve Gastrointestinal Functioning

1. Nutritional replacement

    — Enteral replacement is the artificial means of supplying nutrients into the stomach via a tube ("tube feeding"). Tubes may be placed into the stomach by way of the nose (naso-gastric tube) or directly into the stomach (gastrostomy tube).

        • Care must be taken to correctly place a nasogastric tube so that it is not inadvertently placed into the trachea.

        • A Levine tube is the most common single lumen naso-gastric tube. Small-bore flexible tubes (Vinonex, Dobhoff or Duo) are used for certain types of continuous enteral feedings.

        • A variety of enteral diets are available and prescribed according to the metabolic needs of the individual. For individuals with stable GI function in the home setting, a blenderized regular diet eaten by the rest of the family may be appropriate and well accepted.

        • A continuous slow infusion of hyperosmolar (calorie rich) feedings are tolerated better than bolus or intermittent feedings.

        • Diarrhea is the most common side effect associated with tube feeding. It can be minimized if the feedings are initiated slowly and at half strength. The strength is gradually increased as the GI tract becomes accustomed to the presence of nutrients.

        • For individuals receiving both tube feedings and intravenous lipids, blue food coloring may be added to the tube feeding solution so as not to inadvertently confuse the solutions and for monitoring of aspiration.

    — Parenteral replacement is the mode of supplying nutrients to individuals with nonfunctioning GI tracts or to individuals requiring supplemental nutrients or calories. Solutions may be administered through large lumen peripheral veins or central veins.

        • Total parenteral nutrition (TPN) solutions are primarily high glucose content (25-50%), amino acids, vitamins and trace elements. Lipids may also be administered.

        • Complications of TPN administration may include infection, altered serum glucose levels, fluid overload, elevated CO_2 levels, electrolyte imbalances, and infiltration or dislodging the infusion catheter. Periodic assessment of the serum glucose by fingerstick with supplemental insulin administra-

tion minimizes the pro-blems associated with glucose imbalances. Meticulous care of the infusion site minimizes
secondary, nosocomial infections.

2. Gastric or intestinal decompression

— Tube placement with intermittent suctioning is implemented to
remove accumulated gas and fluid proximal to an obstructed
or injured segment of the tract.

— The purpose of decompression is to remove GI contents because a segment of the tract is obstructed or has ceased functioning adequately (paralytic ileus). The absence of contents
and juices also diminishes peristaltic activity and allows the GI
tract to rest and heal following an injury or surgery.

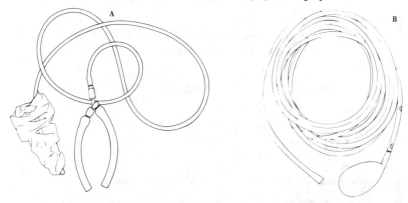

Fig. 4-3. Intestinal tubes: (A) Miller-Abbott tube; (B) Cantor tube. From W.J.
Phipps, B.C. Long, N.F. Woods: _Medical-Surgical Nursing: Concepts and Clinical Prac-
tices_, 5th ed.; St. Louis: Mosby-Year Book, Inc., 1995. Reprinted with permission.

— Knowing the location of the end/tip of the tube is important
when verifying the appropriateness of the secretions being removed.

• Gastric secretions may be periodically tested for acidity
level. Medications may be administered in dosages and frequency (titrated) to maintain a desired pH.

• Gastric secretions normally appear clear or pale yellow.
When blood mixes with gastric secretions, secretions appear brownish with black flecks ("coffee grounds"). Gastric
secretions are very acidic.

• Secretions from the small intestine normally appear pale
green and are very alkaline.

3. Medications
   Several categories of medications may be prescribed to control
   GI symptoms. They often do not cure the underlying cause.

   — Antacids are indicated for the relief of symptoms of gastric hy-
     peracidity and are available as over-the-counter interventions.
     As some antacids contain calcium, they also are used as eco-
     nomical calcium supplements. Some bind with phosphate
     ions and are used for electrolyte management for renal failure.

     • Antacids may interfer with the GI absoprtion of other oral
       medications; e.g. chlordiazepoxide (Librium); isoniazid
       (INH); phenytoin (Dilantin); propranodol (Inderal); barbit-
       urates; digoxin; tetracylclines; and histamine antagonists
       (Tagamet).

     • Antacids may block the autodigestive activity of pancreatic
       enzymes associated with an acute episode of pancreatitis.

   — Histamine H$_2$ receptor antagonists such as cimetidine
     (Tagamet), famotidine (Pepcid), and nizatidine (Axid), reduce
     gastric acid secretions by blocking the action of histamine.

   — Digestive enzyme supplements (Pancreatin, Viokase) require
     specific administration routines to be effective. Usually they
     are taken with food.

   — Peristaltic activity can be modified by medications.

     • Metoclopromide hydrochloride (Reglan) and neostigmine
       (Prostigmin) stimulate peristalsis especially when dimin-
       ished GI activity is slow to return following intestinal sur-
       gery.

     • Antiemetics minimize reverse peristalsis to control nau-
       sea/vomiting; e.g. dimenhydrinate (Dramamine); pro-
       chlorperazine (Compazine); trimethobenzamide HCl
       (Tigan).

     • Anti-diarrheal agents slow large intestine motility; diphe-
       noxylate HCl and Lomotil (atropine).

     • Laxatives augment various normal physiological functions of
       the large intestine, such as retaining water in the contents,
       lubricating contents or increasing peristaltic movement
       through the colon.

4. Surgical correction of the underlying problem may be indicated
   especially when an obstruction is present. The names of the surgical procedures are usually specific to the anatomical structures
   involved and the procedure performed. The impact on physiological function can therefore be easily identified.

Examples:

* Gastrectomy refers to the removal (-ectomy) of the stomach (gastr-).

* Cholycystectomy refers to the removal (-ectomy) of the gall- (choly-) bladder (cys).

* Esophagojejunostomy refers to a surgical opening (-ostomy) made between the esophagus and the jejunum.

* Ileostomy refers to a surgical opening (-ostomy) made into the ileum.

* Colectomy refers to the removal (-ectomy) of the colon or large intestine.

* Surgical by-pass procedures or shunting of hepatic circulation is described by the anatomical names of the involved vessels, e.g. splenorenal shunt refers to the attachment of splenic and renal vessels and a portocaval shunt refers to the attachment of the portal and inferior vena cava veins.

5. Fecal diversion

   – Due to certain obstructive or ulcerative conditions of the large intestine it becomes necessary to surgically create an alternative passage of stool. An artificial opening or stoma is created between the large intestine and the abdominal skin surface.

   – Colostomy is a surgical opening (stoma) anywhere along the colon in which a segment of the large intestine is brought through the abdomen to the surface.

     • Transverse or "loop" colostomy is usually a temporary opening into the transverse colon. It may have two openings and is also called double-barrel colostomy. Soft, unformed stool passes from the proximal stoma and small amounts of mucus are eliminated from the distal opening (mucous fistula). Sometimes a supporting rod is placed beneath the loop to externalize the segment of intestine and stomas until corrective surgery to reconnect intestinal segments (re-anastomosis) can be done.

     • Descending or sigmoid colostomy is usually a permanent diversion with the stoma located on the left side of the abdomen. When the rectum is also removed, the surgical procedure is called abdominoperineal colon resection.

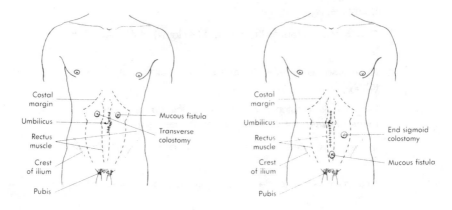

Fig. 4-4. Colostomy sites: *Left, transverse colostomy with adjacent mucous fistula. Right, end sigmoid colostomy and mucous fistula. From W.J. Phipps, B.C. Long, N.F. Woods:* Medical-Surgical Nursing: Concepts and Clinical Practices, *5th ed.; St. Louis: Mosby-Year Book, Inc., 1995. Reprinted with permission.*

- Conventional (Brooke) ileostomy is a permanent diversion of the distal portion of the ileum to the skin surface with the total removal of the colon (colectomy). The continous drainage is liquid and contains digestive enzymes.

- Continent (Kock pouch) ileostomy involves the surgical creation of an intra-abdominal pouch made of the distal segment of the ileum which acts as a reservior. Accumulated intestinal contests are drained 3-4 times a day by inserting a catheter into the reservior through a stoma.

- Ileoanal reservior involves a two-stage surgical creation of intestinal continuity following colectomy. The ileal reservior is constructed between the ileum and the anal canal. Anal spincter control is preserved and bowel control achieved within 3-6 months following reconstructive surgery.

- Teaching about the care of a colostomy or ileostomy begins before surgery by answering questions and drawing pictures to describe the procedure. Self-care teaching begins with the first dressing and pouch change. Viewing the stoma is encouraged and well received when the nurse conveys positive acceptance of the care activities.

  - During the immediate post-operative period the contents of the pouch are monitored for the amount and nature of the drainage. It is not unusal for new ileostomies to drain 1000-1500 ml in a 24-hour period. This volume is calculated as output.

- As peristalsis returns, the pouch may fill with flatus which requires periodic release. An over-inflated pouch may break the skin seal and lead to leakage of contents.

- Care of the skin around the stoma and under the pouch attachment are essential to prevent skin breakdown and infection. The more liquid the drainage, the greater the concern with skin care. Prevention of skin breakdown is easier, less expensive and less painful than any treatment endeavor.

- A closed, sealed system for drainage collection includes a pouch, attachment and skin barrier. Several products which include karaya are available (powder, paste, washer or wafer) to provide a seal between the pouch applicance and the skin surface. Additional information and detailed teaching plans are available from the United Ostomy Association and the American Cancer Society. Many facilities have a clinical nurse specialist (CNS) trained in ostomy care who assists individuals and families to acquire self-care and coordinate discharge planning and follow-up care.

SECTION 3: CLINICAL EXAMPLES OF COMMON GI CONDITIONS

Upper GI Conditions

1. Hiatal hernia (diaphragmatic hernia)
   - A portion of the stomach protrudes upward through the diaphragm into the chest. Conditions associated with increased intra-abdomonal pressure are contributing factors (obesity, pregnancy, ascites).

     - The most common type is a sliding hiatal hernia in which the protrusion and associated symptoms are more pronounced when the individual assumes a supine position. The intensity of symptoms subsides when the person is sitting or standing as the protrusion "slides" back into the abdominal cavity.

   - Reflux of gastric secretions causes heartburn and substernal chest pain. This condition is referred to as GERD (gastroesophageal reflux disease). Belching and regurgitation without nausea occurs. Inflammation and subsequent scarring may result in cardiac stricture which in turn aggravates the symptoms.

- Dilatation of constricted cardiac sphincter may facilitate food passage into the stomach. Surgical repair may be required to restore esophagogastric continuity.

- Dietary management with small meals and limitation of gastric acid stimulating foods minimize the symptoms. Antacids, histamine H_2 receptor blockers and smooth muscle relaxants minimize the reflux esophagitis.

- Place the individual's bed in a trendelenburg position to promote comfort while sleeping.

2. Gastric (peptic) and duodenal ulcers.

  - Many cases of peptic ulcer disease are associated with an infection caused by Helicobacter pylori.

  - Increased acidity or stasis of gastric secretions may lead to erosion of the stomach mucosa (peptic ulcer) or the mucosa of the first segment of the small intestine (duodenal ulcer).

    - A high-stress lifestyle, smoking, irritating medications and other disease processes are known contributory factors. Also, prolonged stress from severe burn injury or trauma can produce ulcers. With non-surgical treatment, most ulcers heal within 4-6 weeks.

    - Caffeine, alcohol consumption, steroids, salicylates, reserpine, indomethacin and anti-inflammatory agents aggravate sensitive GI mucosa.

    - Inflammation of the pancreas and/or the liver is associated with increased gastric secretion and subsequent ulcer formation.

  - A characteristic symptom is epigastric ("burning") pain between meals and at night when the stomach is empty. Eating often minimizes duodenal ulcer pain but aggravates peptic ulcer pain.

  - Conservative management includes dietary modification to avoid caffeine liquids and to eat regular, nutritionally balanced meals. Protein in the stomach acts as a natural buffer for gastric acid and slows the movement of gastric contents into the duodenum.

    - Antacids are prescribed for symptom relief by neutralizing the gastric acidity (increasing the gastric pH).

    - Histamine H_2 receptor blockers (cimetidine/Tagamet, ranitidine/Zantac, famotidine/Pepcid) suppress the secretion of gastric acid and thereby facilitate healing. It is important that these medications be taken with meals (or 1 hour before) and at bedtime as 60% of gastric secretions occur at night.

- Sucralfate (Carafate) coats the ulcer with a protective barrier which prevents further irritation and allows healing to occur.

- Gastric secretions may also be titrated with antacid administration via nasogastric intubation. After 60-90 ml are instilled, the tube is clamped for 20-30 minutes. The pH of the gastric contents is re-assessed. Antacid administration is repeated until the pH is greater than 4.5.

- Appropriate antibiotic therapy is required for _H. pylori_ infections. The drugs of choice for organism eradication include Rantitidine plus Bismuth subsalicytate tablets, Metronidazole and tetracycline. Other antibiotics may be substituted if specific drug allergy is present.

— When an ulcer bleeds, characteristic changes occur to the blood. If active bleeding occurs at the esophagogastric junction, the emesis is bright red. If the blood mixes with gastric secretions, the blood appears like "coffee grounds." Blood that passes through the intestinal tract changes stool to a black tarry appearance (melena).

— The majority of ulcers heal by non-surgical interventions, however, surgical intervention is performed when ulceration results in hemorrhage, obstruction or perforation. Bleeding occurs in about 15-20% of persons with ulcers and rebleeding occurs in 25-40% of these persons. About 10% of ulcers perforate with subsequent peritonitis.

- Pyloroplasty enlarges the pyloric sphincter to relieve obstructive scarring.

- Vagotomy refers to the severing of a branch of the vagus nerve to inhibit gastric acid secretion.

- Gastrectomy is the removal of a portion of the stomach with attachment (anastomosis) of the remaining stomach to the duodenum (gastroduodenostomy) or jejunum (gastrojejunostomy). Decreased production of intrinsic factor resulting in secondary pernicious anemia may occur following a total gastrectomy.

— When a large portion of the stomach is removed, there is a risk for contents to move very quickly into the small intestine ("dumping syndrome"). Symptoms of weakness, diaphoresis, tachycardia and dizziness may occur. Small, low-carbohydrate feedings with minimal liquids minimize this problem.

Small Intestine Conditions

1. Crohn's Disease (regional enteritis)

— This inflammatory disease affects any segment of the GI tract with the terminal ileum being the most frequently involved site. Inflamed areas of the intestine are located between uninvolved segments. The intensity and severity of involvement and symptoms vary. The etiology is unknown; however, infection, immunologic factors and genetic predisposition are contributing factors.

— Onset of symptoms may be sudden, resembling acute appendicitis or ulcerative colitis. Unexplained diarrhea with colic or cramping is the most common clinical manifestation. Colic pain is relieved by bowel movement.

  • Intestinal, digestive enzymes often are lost in the diarrhea, causing undigested fat in the stool (steatorrhea). Fat-soluble vitamins (A, D, E and K) are poorly absorbed.

  • Stool examination reveals occult blood. Frank blood is present in the stool when the lower colon is involved. Stool cultures rule out bacterial or parasitic causes.

— Barium enema and direct visualization by colonoscopy rule out other causes and identify the extent of the inflammatory involvement.

— During acute episodes, treatment focuses on minimizing the acuity of symptoms with sulfasalazine, corticosteroids, and replacing fluids and electrolytes. Antidiarrheal preparations may be prescribed to decrease intestinal motility and cramping. Pain management narcotics, such as Demoral, may be indicated for severe abdominal pain.

  • Surgical intervention is performed only if intestinal obstruction, abscesses or perforation occurs. Removal of involved segments is not a cure.

2. Obstructive processes

Obstruction of the small intestine involves conditions in which the peristaltic movement of intestinal contents is impaired or totally blocked.

— Paralytic ileus is the cessation of peristalsis as a result of impaired neural impulse transmission. General anesthesia, direct irritation or manipulation of the gastrointestinal tissues (GI surgery) are the most common causes.

  • When peristalsis ceases, the proximal segment becomes distended from accumulated food, secretions and gas. Re-

Focused Bedside Assessment

There is the possibility that an intestinal condition may worsen, causing leakage of intestinal contents into the peritoneal cavity. As intestinal juices are very irritating to surrounding tissue, the early identification of peritonitis minimizes the development of a more serious complication (sepsis). The following assessment data are associated with the early development of peritonitis or "acute abdomen" which warrants prompt notification of the physician.

* **General appearance**: Malaise, fever, weakness, abdominal pain.

* **Neurological status**: Restless; otherwise WNL.

* **Cardiac status**: Tachycardia due to inflammation and possible septic shock; otherwise WNL.

* **Respiratory status**: Tachcyapnea due to inflammation and possible shock; lung sounds WNL.

* **Abdominal (GI) status**: Taut distention; abdomen becomes more firm ("rigid" or "board-like"); increasing local or diffuse abdominal pain; decreased to absent bowel sounds; nausea/vomiting, change in bowel elimination pattern.

* **Urinary elimination status**: WNL and appropriate for fluid intake unless septic shock is developing. Diminishing urinary output, in spite of adequate fluid intake, warrants further assessment.

* **Extremities**: All peripheral pulses are present. Warm, dry extremities, elevated body temperature with a warm chest and abdomen may suggest an infection. (Remember that elderly persons may normally have below normal body temperatures.) If the extremities are cool, clammy and diaphoretic with a warm chest and abdomen further assessment is warranted.

* When the individual is turned to their side, the nurse would expect to assess no unusual findings.

If additional data are observed, a more detailed assessment of the involved system is required. Additional areas of physiological dysfunction may be present and confound the present "acute abdomen" problem.

verse peristalsis (vomiting) is a natural attempt to relieve the distention.

Refer to GI physiology for additional information on potential volume of GI secretions produced daily.

* Clinical manifestations include bloated feeling, observable distention with tympani, decreased bowel sounds and no passage of stool or flatus.

- Gastrointestinal decompression is initiated until bowel sounds return. Metoclopramide hydrochloride (Reglan) or neostigmine (Prostigmin) may be prescribed to stimulate peristaltic activity.

- As distention continues, the intestinal wall becomes inflamed with subsequent impaired circulation. Rupture and peritonitis may occur.

— Small bowel obstruction may result from various mechanical causes. Repeated inflammatory episodes may cause scar tissue (adhesions) which constricts the internal intestinal opening and passage of contents. Increased peristaltic activity proximal to a narrowed segment may twist (volvulus) or telescope within itself (intussusception).

- Intestinal obstruction may also occur with persons who have a history of a neoplasm within the abdominal cavity. Extension or metastasis to surrounding structures may compress or occlude segments of the intestine.

- A blood clot may develop in a mesenteric vein which supplies the intestine (mesenteric thrombosis) causing a vascular infarction and subsequent gangrenous segment of the intestine. The onset of vascular obstructive symptoms is abrupt with rapidly developing signs of hypovolemic shock.

3. Hernia
   — Any protrusion of an organ from its normal cavity into an adjacent cavity is termed a hernia. Most commonly a loop of intestine passes through the abdominal wall. When the loop cannot be manipulated back into the abdominal cavity, it is termed irreducible or incarcerated. If the blood supply is impaired, the hernia is termed strangulated.

   - An inguinal hernia occurs when a loop of the intestine descends along the inguinal canal into the scrotum or labia. While a femoral hernia occurs in the same general anatomical area, the intestinal loop descends through the same opening for the femoral artery and femoral vein.

   - An umbilical hernia is a protrusion of intestinal loop which everts the umbilicus. This type of hernia rarely causes physiological problems.

   - An incisional hernia is a protrusion of intestinal loop through an old surgical incision in which the skin surface remains intact. This type of hernia is not to be confused with a wound separation (dehiscence) or a protrusion of intestine through a new incision (evisceration).

— Surgical repair (herniorrhaphy or hernioplasty) is the only cure for a hernia and is often performed in ambulatory surgical services. Occasionally this condition is present in persons whose frail or unstable physical condition does not permit surgical repair. In these situations, assessment of the adequacy of intestinal function and blood supply to involved structures is important for the early identification of potential complications.

Large Intestine Conditions

1. Cancer of the bowel (colorectal cancer)

   — Malignant tumors of the colon and rectum are among the most common malignancies in the United States. The incidence increases with age. Surgical removal with restoration of GI continuity is the primary treatment.

   — Cleansing preparation of the bowel begins several days before surgery with the use of enemas and antibiotics to reduce the normal bacterial growth in the colon. Neomycin and/or erythromycin preparations are commonly prescribed.

   — Surgical removal (resection) of the lesion and surrounding segment of colon is the treatment. For lesions above the rectum, the remaining segment of colon is attached (anastomosed) to the rectum through an abdominal incision.

     • When the rectum is involved, it is removed through a wide perineal excision. The remaining segment of the descending colon is brought to the surface of the left side of the abdomen. A permanent colostomy is formed. The perineal incision is packed with gauze and drains to facilitate healing from the inside toward the surface. Meticulous wound care prevents secondary infections.

     • Chemotherapy and/or radiation are administered in combination with surgical resection.

2. Colitis

   — Chronic inflammation of the large intestine usually begins in the rectosigmoid segment and may progress proximally to involve the entire large intestine. Inflamed areas lead to ulceration and possible perforation and fistula formation between intestinal walls. Open lesions may become infected forming abscesses.

     • The irritation from the inflammatory process causes varying degrees of diarrhea with fluid and electrolyte loss. It is not unusual for a person with acute ulcerative colitis to have 15-

20 liquid stools daily that contain undigested food, intestinal fluid, blood, mucus and pus.

- If the inflammatory process cannot be controlled by medication and nutritional support, the removal of the colon (total colectomy) and a permanent ileostomy are performed.

3. Diverticulum

   — Small outpouching or sacs of mucosal tissue are formed through the muscle layer of the large intestine. The occurrence increases with age and is asymptomatic unless a sac becomes inflamed (diverticulitis). An adequate intake of dietary fiber minimizes the collection of intestinal contents in diverticular sacs thus averting an acute inflammatory response.

   - An acute episode is usually self-limiting with intestinal rest, fluid replacement and antibiotic therapy. Recurrent episodes or abscess formation may require resection of the involved colon or temporary colon diversion (double-barrel colostomy).

4. Hemorrhoids

   — The veins in the rectal area become congested and may thrombose in a manner similar to varicose veins in other locations. Conditions associated with prolonged, increased intra-abdominal pressure are likely to result in distended rectal veins.

   - Care during rectal procedures and prevention of constipation will minimize problems for persons hospitalized for the treatment of other, non-related conditions.

   - Recurring episodes of bleeding or thrombosed hemorrhoids may be treated by ligation or injection of sclerosing solution in ambulatory surgical services.

Accessory Digestive Conditions

1. Galbladder Disease - Inflamatory and/or stones.

   — Cholelithiasis refers to the presence of stones in the gallbladder. Cholecystitis refers to the inflammation of the gallbladder. The incidence of these conditions accounts for a major reason for hospitalization and surgery for adults.

   - High-risk factors include obesity; middle age; medical history of diabetes mellitus, endocrine dysfunction or liver disease; females receiving birth control medication; persons with high serum cholesterol levels.

- The primary clinical symptom of an acute episode includes sudden onset of mid-epigastric pain, which may radiate to the right shoulder, following the ingestion of high-caloric food. The pain is often intense and associated with tachycardia, diaphoresis, nausea and vomiting.

If the duct leading to the duodenum is obstructed, the absence of bile causes clay-colored stools. The bile flow will back up into the liver and eventually into the blood causing jaundice.

- Surgical intervention is often required to restore bile flow and digestion. Several different procedures are possible depending upon the stone location and anatomical involvement.

  • Lithotripsy involves the disintegration of small stones by using ultrasonic sound waves. Often this procedure is accomplished with only a brief hospitalization or as an outpatient procedure.

  • Cholecystectomy refers to the removal of the gallbladder, whereas, choledocholithotomy refers to the removal of astone from the common bile duct.

  • A laprascopic cholecystectomy requires hospitalization for one day and most individuals return to work within one week. An abdominal cholecystectomy may require a hospital stay of four to five days with a recovery time of six weeks.

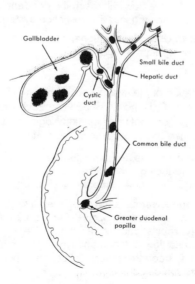

Fig. 4-5. **Common sites of gallstones.** _From W.J. Phipps, B.C. Long, N.F. Woods: Medical-Surgical Nursing: Concepts and Clinical Practices, 5th ed.; St. Louis: Mosby-Year Book, Inc., 1995. Reprinted with permission._

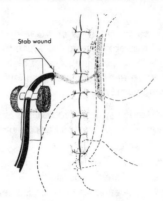

Stab wound

Fig. 4-6. Section of T-tube. From W.J. Phipps, B.C. Long, N.F. Woods: Medical-Surgical Nursing, 5th ed.; St. Louis: Mosby-Year Book, Inc., 1995. Reprinted with permission.

— If the common bile duct is incised, a T-tube is placed in the duct with the long end of the tube extending through the abdominal skin surface. This tube is placed to preserve patency of the duct and bile flow until the post-operative edema has subsided. Excess bile flows by gravity to a closed collection device (Duvol or Jackson-Pratt).

  • During the immediate post-operative period, the amount of drainage may reach 500-1000 ml/24 hours. Within 5-7 days, the bile flow will reach the duodenum with no excess drainage flowing into the collection system.

  • Refer to Unit 8 for additional information on post-operative care and pain management.

2. Hepatitis
   — Inflammation of the liver is caused by one of the hepatitis viruses (A, B, C, D, non-A or non-B). Each virus is related to specific immunologic and epidemiologic factors. Regardless of the cause, the symptomology is similar.

  • When liver cells are damaged, abnormal liver function occurs producing characteristic clinical manifestations and changes in specific laboratory tests.

  • Damaged liver cells have regenerative capability. However, when necrosis occurs, fibrous replacement and scarring (cirrhosis) causes permanent liver dysfunction and disrupted flow of blood and lymph through the liver. Depending upon the severity of scarring, hepatic failure and death may result.

  • It is estimated that 20% of cases of hepatitis develop permanent liver damage (postnecrotic cirrhosis).

Focused Bedside Assessment

The following assessment data would be expected during the immediate post-operative period following an abdominal cholecystectomy. No other pathophysiological problems involving other body system dysfunction unrelated to gallbladder disease and related post-operative care is included.

* **General appearance:** Awakens easily; oriented; readily returns to sleeping state for the first 48 hours post-op; post-operative pain well managed with PCA infusion or regular injections.

* **Neurological status:** WNL.

* **Cardiac status:** WNL; tachycardia may be present with acute incisional pain.

* **Respiratory status:** Incisional pain may cause shallow ventilations; diaphragmatic irritation may cause referred pain to the right shoulder. Incentive inspirometry equal 2X normal inspiratory effort. For example, the tidal volume (TV or normal breath) equals 8-10ml/KG of body weight. For a person weighing 135# or 61 Kg, the TV = 480-610 ml/breath, deep breathing equals 2X TV or 960-1220 ml/breath.

* **Abdominal (GI) status:** Decreased bowel sounds; as peristalsis returns belching decreases; return of passing flatus indicates that peristalsis is WNL; stool resumes normal color as bile reaches the small intestine; no drainage on the dressing; abdomen soft.

* **Urinary elimination status:** WNL and appropriate for fluid intake.

* **Extremities:** Peripheral pulses WNL; movement WNL.

* When the individual is turned on their side, the nurse would expect to assess no unusual findings

If additional data are observed, a more detailed assessment of the involved system is required. Additional areas of physiological dysfunction may be present and confound the present clinical situation.

— Jaundice is the predominant symptom associated with decreased liver function. It occurs with rapid breakdown of red blood cells (hemolytic), increased production of bilirubin, dysfunctioning liver cells (hepatocellular), or an obstruction in the flow of bile from the liver (posthepatic obstructive).

  • Additional symptoms include nausea, vomiting, malaise, fatigue, epigastric abdominal pain, dark ("cola" colored) urine, clay-colored stool and itching (pruritus).

— Diagnosis is determined by identifying immunological markers specific to Hepatitis A and Hepatitis B; elevated liver enzymes (SGOT, SGPT); elevated bilirubin levels; prolonged prothrom-

Focused Bedside Assessment

The following data are expected during an acute episode of hepatitis. No other pathophysiological problems involving non-related body system dysfunction is included.

* **General appearance**: Malaise, weakness, low-grade fever; jaundice.

* **Neurological status**: WNL unless ammonia is being retained. Increased lethargy and sleeping with difficulty in arousing and poor orientation warrant further assessment.

* **Cardiac status**: WNL unless portal hypertension is developing. Increasing blood pressure and clinical manifestations of congestive heart failure warrant further assessment. Soft tissue bruising from minimal injury may indicate impaired bleeding/clotting response.

* **Respiratory status**: WNL unless cardiovascular function is compromised or abdominal distention is present. Increasing dyspnea with minimal exertion or noctural dyspnea warrant further assessment.

* **Abdominal (GI) status**: Soft, distention; tenderness to pain in the right upper quadrant; liver may be palpated below the right rib cage. If portal hypertension develops, the abdominal cavity may become filled with fluid (ascites).

* **Urinary elimination status**: The volume is WNL. As bile pigments may be excreted in the urine, the color may become darker. Urine may be assessed for the pressence of protein which may indicate increased capillary permeability within the kidneys.

* **Extremities**: WNL unless a fluid retention problem develops.

* When the individual is turned on their side, the nurse would expect to assess no unusual findings.

If additional data are observed, a more detailed assessment of the involved system is required. Additional areas of physiological dysfunction may be present and confound the present clinical situation.

bin time (PT). WBC differential count will indicate elevated leukocytes, monocytes and atypical lymphocytes.

— Management of care focused on controlling symptoms and minimizing liver dysfunction.

   • Physical rest is important to minimize the metabolic requirements. Gamma globulin injections are administered to personal contacts to prevent transmission of the virus.

   • Sodium and protein intake is restricted to only daily requirements. All alcoholic beverages are strictly avoided.

- Vitamin K (mephyton, menadione) is administered when the prothrombin time (PT) is prolonged. Other measures to minimize tissue injury or bleeding are implemented; e.g. soft-bristle toothbrush, electric razors.

- Observe for side effects and toxicity of medications as chemical breakdown (detoxification) is slowed, delaying the release of active ingredients into circulation. Due to altered drug metabolism, longer time may be required to achieve therapeutic levels or active ingredients may remain longer in circulation.

- Numerous medications are known to be hepatotoxic and should be avoided as they may cause further liver impairment. Other preparations can usually be substituted for the desired action.

Table 4-1. Common Hepatotoxic Drugs

Generic/category name	Common trade names
acetaminophen	Tylenol
acetylsalicylic acid	Aspirin
ampicillin	Omnipen, Polycillin, Pfizerpen A
carbamazepine	Tegretol
carbenicillin	Geopen, Pyopen
chlorpropamide	Diabinese
chlorpromazine	Thorazine
cindamycin	Cleocin
diazepam	Valium
hydrochlorothiazide	Esidrix
ospmoazod	Isotamine
methyldopa	Aldomet
oral contraceptives	
oxacillin	Bactocill
penicillin	Pen-Vee K, Pfizerpen VK
phenytoin sodium	Dilantin
propylthiouracil (PTU)	Propyl-Thyracil
rifampin	Rifadin
sulfonamides	Bactrim, Septra, Gantrisin
tetracyclines (especially parenteral)	Achromycin

Adapted from P.L. Swearingen: Manual of Medical-Surgical Nursing, *3rd ed.; St. Louis: Mosby-Year Book, Inc., 1994.*

3. Liver failure

   — Initially, the size of the liver increases (hepatomegaly). With the majority of liver function impaired, the flow of blood and lymph is impaired causing further pathophysiological changes in adjacent structures.

- The backup or congestion within the vascular system leads to portal hypertension and distended veins in the esophagus (esophageal varies) and in the rectum (hemorrhoids). Spontaneous bleeding from varices may be life-threatening.

- The increased intravascular pressure causes capillary permeability and movement of fluid and plasma proteins out of the vessels into the surrounding tissue and body cavities: interstitial edema and ascites. Diuretics such as aldosterone antagonists or loop diuretics may be used to alleviate edema. Paracentesis may also be used to treat ascites.

  − The process of damage causing more damage becomes cyclic. For example, if bleeding occurs due to injury to esophageal varies or prolonged prothrombin times, the liver is unable to convert the products of damaged red blood cells. Thus, increasing injury to liver cells occurs.

  - A similar cyclic process develops with metabolism of protein. Ammonia, a product of protein metabolism, accumulates in the blood. This substance is very toxic to brain tissue causing hepatic encephalopathy (hepatic coma). Varying signs of mental confusion and lethargy may be observed as serum ammonia (NH_3) increases.

  - Cephulac (lactulose) is prescribed orally or by retention enema to bind with the ammonia ions and facilitate intestinal excretion.

4. Pancreatitis
   − When the pancreas becomes inflamed exocrine (digestive enzyme) and endocrine (insulin production) activities are affected. Initially, the pancreatic ducts become occluded and the pancreatic enzymes do not reach the small intestine in adequate amounts. Fat and protein digestion is ineffective leading to malabsorption, fluid and electrolyte loss. As the process continues, the beta cells become damaged, decreasing insulin production, resulting in secondary diabetes mellitus.

     - Ingested food provides the stimulus for pancreatic enzyme excretion. When an inflamed pancreas is unable to produce an adequate flow into the small intestine, enzymes (amylase, lipase and trypsin) begin to react with surrounding pancreatic tissue (autodigestion). The inflammatory process is extended, causing hemorrhage and necrosis. As the inflammatory process accelerates, the sequence becomes cyclic.

- Acute pancreatitis is characterized by sudden onset of severe epigastric pain and persistent vomiting after eating a large meal or ingesting alcohol. Signs of shock may develop rapidly especially in an elderly person. Hypotension, tachycardia, pulmonary congestion, diaphoresis and restlessness are observed.

- Elevated serum amylase and lipase levels confirm the diagnosis and reflect the degree of necrotic pancreatic tissue. Elevated WBC count confirms the inflammatory process. The presence of polymorphonuclear bodies suggests an associated secondary bacterial peritonitis.

  • Hyperglycemia with acidosis is present when the beta cells are involved. Supplemental insulin administration may be required to stabilize the glucose imbalance.

- Management of an acute episode includes pain management with the liberal use of meperidine (Demerol). Morphine and derivatives tend to increase sphincter spasms and may contribute to obstructed pancreatic ducts.

  • The gastrointestinal tract is placed at rest to decrease the stimulation of enzyme excretion. Until the inflammatory process subsides the following measures are implemen-ted: nasogastric intubation with low continuous via Salem sump suction; intravenous fluid and electrolyte replacement, and hyperalimentation for nutritional requirements. Pharmacologic therapy includes use of antacids to neutralize gastric secretion or histamine antagonists to lower gastric acid production. In chronic cases, replacement pancreatic enzymes may be indicated.

  • Localized areas of necrotic tissue or pancreatic cysts may be surgically incised and drained. Bleeding is surgically controlled when hemorrhagic pancreatitis is localized. As the surgical risk is very high in these situations, the immediate post-operative period is usually monitored in a critical care setting.

unit *5*

NURSING CARE OF ADULTS WITH

Metabolic/Reproductive Conditions

T*his unit addresses a variety of commonly recurring conditions of adults which affect the physiological functioning of the endocrine and/or reproductive systems. The care of individuals with uncomplicated metabolic and/or reproductive dysfunction on general medical-surgical nursing units is addressed. The management and care of critical and unstable clinical situations, which require continuous monitoring, are usually cared for in specialty care units and are not included in this unit. Examples of clinical conditions requiring high acuity care include acute diabetic keto-acidosis (DKA), hyperosmolar hyperglycemic non-ketotic coma (HHNC), insulin shock, thyrotoxic crisis and adrenal (Addisonian) crisis.*

SECTION 1: OVERVIEW

Effective plans for care are based upon an understanding of the normal functioning of the endocrine and reproductive systems. These body systems are composed of the several glands and organs which work together with the central nervous system to coordinate an optimal internal environment for physiological functioning. This interrelated response is accomplished by the stimulation and release of chemical substances (hormones) into the general circulation of blood and body fluids. Each hormone has a specific action(s) which directly affects selected receptors or target cells in the body.

Anatomical Considerations

1. The endocrine system is composed of the pituitary gland, thyroid, parathyroids, adrenals, Islet cells of the pancreas, ovaries and testes. The pineal, hypothalamus and thymus glands are included in this system but are not discussed in this unit.

    — The pituitary gland is known as the master gland because its secretions affect other glands. It is located at the base of the skull in a protective bony depression called the sella tursica. It has two distinctly separate lobes: anterior pituitary and the posterior pituitary.

    — The thyroid gland is located in the anterior portion of the neck just below the larynx. Two pairs of parathyroid glands are located on the posterior side of the thyroid gland.

    — The adrenal glands are located just superior to each kidney. Each gland is composed of two portions -- the inner medulla and the outer cortex.

       • The adrenal medulla accounts for 20% of the weight of the gland. It secretes catecholamines (epinephrine and norepinephrine) and dopamine which are integral to an effective stress response.

       • The adrenal cortex accounts for 80% of the weight of the gland. It produces aldosterone and glucocorticoid (steroid) hormones.

    — The endocrine pancreas consists of the islet (beta) cells which are located throughout the gland. They secrete glucagon and insulin into the general circulation to regulate carbohydrate, protein and fat metabolism.

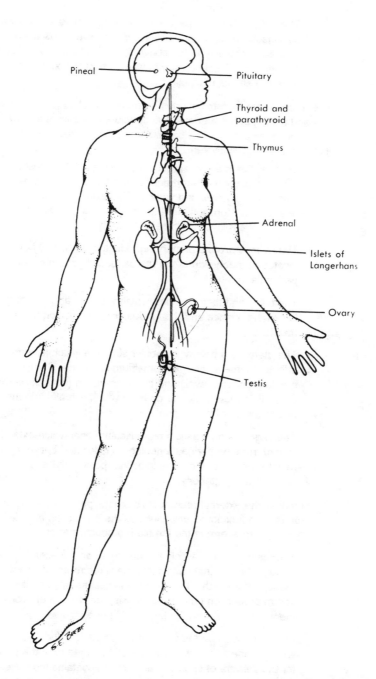

Fig. 5-1. Endocrine system. _From S.M. Tucker, et. al.: Patient Care Standards, 6th ed.; St. Louis: Mosby-Year Book, Inc., 1996. Reprinted with permission._

- The beta cells of the pancreas specifically make or synthesize insulin which works closely with the liver, muscles and adipose (fat) tissue in the conversion of nutrients for cellular metabolism. Glucagon works with cortisol to counterbalance the effects of insulin.

2. The reproductive system includes hormone secreting glands (ovaries and testes) and the anatomical structures for sexual activity and fetal development. The breasts (mammary glands) are also included in this body system.

   — In females, the internal reproductive organs are the most important and essential to reproduction. They are the ovaries, fallopian tubes, uterus and vagina. The external genitalia have accessory functions for the protection of the vaginal opening and are involved in sexual activity.

     - The ovaries are the primary reproductive organs. They are located on each side of the uterus, outside and beneath the peritoneal cavity.

     - The fallopian tubes provide passage for ova and sperm between the ovaries and the fundus or upper portion of the uterus.

     - The uterus is a hallow, muscular structure which is comprised of three layers: endometrium (inner lining), myometrium (muscle layer) and the perimetrium (covering). The cervix is the lower uterine opening which extends into the upper portion of the vagina.

     - The vagina is an elastic, fibromuscular canal which extends inward from the perineal opening. It is located between the rectal segment of the large intestine (posteriorly) and the urinary urethra (anteriorly).

   — In males, the external reproductive organs perform the major reproductive functions, which include the production and delivery of mature sperm in the female reproductive tract.

     - The testes develop within the abdomen and descend through the inguinal canals into the scrotum about one month before birth. This descent is necessary because sperm production (spermatogenesis) requires an environment 2-3 degrees cooler than body temperature.

     - The epididymis and vas deferens comprise a duct system which connects the testes to the urinary urethra in the penis for the delivery of sperm. The scrotum contains the testes, epididymis, vas deferens and spermatic cord.

• The penis contains the urethra and vascular spaces which become engorged during sexual stimulation.

• The internal male reproductive organs include glands and ducts which produce secretions to promote sperm motility and survival. The sperm and fluids are called semen. The prostate gland, which surrounds the urethra at the base of the urinary bladder, is the major producer of seminal fluid.

Normal Physiological Functioning

1. Endocrine system

  — The two primary hormones secreted by the posterior pituitary gland are antidiuretic hormone (ADH) and oxytocin. The release of these hormones is triggered by selected sympathetic nervous system impulses.

    • ADH or vasopressin acts on the kidneys to retain sodium, to increase the water reabsorption and to concentrate the urine. These actions result in an increase or restoration of arterial blood pressure when it has fallen to a dangerously low level.

    • High doses of ADH (vasopressin) may be administered topically to achieve hemostasis for localized hemorrhage.

    • Oxytocin is responsible for uterine contractions and lactation in females. It is released in response to suckling at the breast and distention of the uterus. It has an antidiuretic effect similar to ADH in both men and women.

  — The hormones secreted by the anterior pituitary gland are:

    • Adrenocorticotropic hormone (ACTH) which stimulates activity of the adrenal glands.

    • Melanocyte-stimulating hormone (MSH) which stimulates the secretion of melanin for skin pigmentation.

    • Somatotropic or growth hormone (GH) which stimulates the bone and muscles for increased growth.

    • Prolactin which stimulates the production of milk in the breast.

    • Thyroid-stimulating hormone (TSH) which stimulates the secretion of thyroid hormone and iodine uptake in the thyroid gland.

- • Follicle stimulating (FSH) and luteninzing hormones (LH) which stimulate the maturation of ovarian follicles and regulate the production of mature sperm.

— The thyroid gland and thyroxine hormone control metabolic processes throughout the body, whereas the parathyroid glands regulate serum calcium levels.

- • Thyroid stimulating hormone (TSH) secreted by the anterior pituitary gland triggers the production of thyroid hormone, thyroxine and prostaglandins by the thyroid gland. Low serum iodine levels will also trigger hormone (TSH) production.

- • Parathyroid glands secrete parathyroid hormone (PTH) along with calcitonin to regulate serum calcium levels. Initially, an increase in serum calcium levels is achieved by increased gastrointestinal absorption of calcium. If this is not sufficient, then breakdown or resorption of bone occurs.

- • Serum magnesium and phosphate levels also trigger parathyroid response and affect serum calcium levels.

— The secretions from the cortex of the adrenal gland have widespread effects on physiological functioning.

- • The steroid hormones, glucocorticoids, secreted by the adrenal cortex affect many physiological functions. These hormones increase blood glucose levels by stimulating glucose formation (gluconeogenesis). They also stimulate protein breakdown (catabolism).

- • Steroid hormones act at several sites in the body to inhibit immune and inflammatory reactions. In addition, they increase the number of circulating erythrocytes, increase appetite, promote fat deposits in the face and neck and decrease serum calcium levels. They enhance the effects of catecholamines, thyroid hormone and growth hormone.

- • Cortisol is the most potent, naturally-occurring glucocorticoid. ACTH triggers its secretion and release into the circulation. Stress has been shown to increase ACTH secretion thus leading to increased cortisol levels.

— Islet (beta) cells of the pancreas produce insulin and glucagon. Insulin is actively involved in the conversion of nutrients into their simplest chemical structure so that they are available for cellular metabolism. Glucagon acts in an opposing manner by converting nutrients into more complex forms for storage and use later.

2. Female Reproductive system

   — The ovaries function in concert with the anterior pituitary gland in the maturation of ova and the secretion of estrogen and progesterone. The inner lining of the uterus (endometrium) responds to hormonal secretions during the menstrual cycle and during pregnancy.

   — The vaginal canal is protected from many infections by the normal population of harmless resident bacteria *(Lactobacillus acidophilus)* and adequate estrogen levels. Antibiotic therapy for systemic infections may alter the normal bacterial growth in the vagina resulting in secondary infections.

   — The female breast develops in response to estrogen secretion. Its primary function is to provide a source of nourishment for the newborn. Lactation also suppresses ovarian activity, menstrual cycle and the release of ova.

     • The anatomical structure of the male breast is similar but, in the absence of high-circulating estrogen levels, does not develop.

Variations Related to Aging

1. The Islets cells of the pancreas tend to decrease in their effectiveness and insulin production. The incidence of age-related glucose intolerance and periodic hyperglycemia increases with aging. Blood glucose levels of an elderly person tend to be slightly above normal and remain elevated somewhat longer after eating as compared to younger non-diabetic adults. Non-insulin-dependent diabetes mellitus (NIDDM) is a common chronic condition among the elderly.

2. Theories of stress and adaptation suggest that the body wears out from overuse and no longer is able to adapt to the cumulative effect of physiological stress. This theory may explain why some elders have decreased ability to respond to the stressors associated with serious illness. Physiological adaptability varies and seems to be an individual response rather than predictable by chronological age.

3. Thyroid function decreases with age resulting in an increasing tendency toward a lower metabolic rate and hypothyroidism. This response accounts for an elder's frequent complaints of being cold, increased sleeping patterns, low body temperature and weight gain.

4. Although the size of the adrenal and pituitary glands decrease, their function does not seem to be affected.

5. Menopause is the normal decline in ovarian function which occurs in women at age 50-55. Transient vasomotor flushes accompanied by dizziness, headaches, palpitations, diaphoresis and/or insomnia are reported by 75-80% of all menopausal women.

    — Urogenital changes occur. The vaginal epithelium atrophies leading to irritation, itching (pruritus) or bleeding. The pH increases altering the normal protective bacterial population leading to increased incidence of infections. The muscle tone relaxes throughout the pelvic area leading to urinary elimination difficulties.

    — Loss of bone mass increases leading to brittleness and porosity which predisposes some women to pathologic bone fractures. Estrogen replacement therapy, weight-bearing exercise, cessation of smoking and increasing calcium intake diminish the development of osteoporosis.

    — Serum cholesterol and triglyceride levels increase with menopause and lowered estrogen levels. Therefore, there is an increased risk for coronary artery disease in women after age 55.

6. Males maintain reproductive capacity longer than females. There is no known discrete event that denotes specific changes in the male reproductive system or ability. Male reproductive functions and hormone secretion diminish with age but do not cease in healthy men. Erectile response may be slower but the sperm count usually remains normal.

    — Reduced testosterone levels cause some loss of function of internal organs and enlargement (hypertrophy) of the prostate gland. Other systemic changes related to aging such as atherosclerosis impact on male reproductive function and sexual capability.

SECTION 2: METABOLIC/ REPRODUCTIVE DYSFUNCTION

Overview

Alterations in the functioning of the endocrine system are usually related to the hypersecretion of hormones (excess) or hyposecretion of hormones (deficit). When an endocrine gland is overstimulated and excess amounts of the hormone are released into circulation, the physiological functioning of that gland is exaggerated. In a comparable manner, when an endocrine gland is understimulated and deficient amounts of hormone are in circulation, the physiological functioning of that gland is impaired.

Assessment of Endocrine (Metabolic) Status

Changes in endocrine function are subtle and often go undetected until serious dysfunction is present. An overlap of symptoms which mimic dysfunction of another body system further complicates an accurate assessment and early diagnosis. The presence of the following symptoms are indicators of an endocrine imbalance and require a more complete evaluation.

1. As endocrine function is associated with metabolic activity, changes in the following physical characteristics may be clues to an underlying endocrine imbalance.

   — Change in body hair texture or distribution especially on the face. Hirsutism refers to excess body hair.

   — Exophthalmus or wide open, protruding stare may be associated with altered thyroid activity.

   — Temperature intolerance and below normal body temperature.

   — Increased incidence or onset of acne in adults and changes in skin pigmentation.

2. Increased incidence of nonserious infections may be associated with altered immune response. When frequent minor infections are also accompanied by environmental temperature intolerance, a more extensive endocrine assessment is warranted.

3. Weight gain or loss not related to fluid and nutritional intake is common with endocrine imbalances. For example, fluid retention and interstitial edema may be associated with a sodium imbalance secondary to impaired adrenal function.

4. Changes in elimination patterns are closely associated with an underlying change in water and electrolyte balance. A history should include information on the frequency, amount and color of urinary elimination. The cause of nocturia (voiding during the night) or dysuria (difficulty or painful urination) should be identified.

   — The classic symptoms of decreased endocrine function of the pancreas (diabetes mellitus) are polyuria (increased urination), polydipsia (increased thirst), and polyphagia (increased appetite).

5. Energy level is a reflection of the underlying metabolic state. Changes may be subtle and go undetected by the individual until serious imbalance is present. Tiredness, weakness and general malaise are common subjective symptoms.

   — When energy level changes accompany altered body temperature or intolerance of environmental temperature, an endocrine imbalance may be present.

6. Altered reproductive function is initially exhibited as altered menstrual cycle or impotence (decreased ability to perform sexually).

7. Electrolyte imbalances may occur with endocrine dysfunction. For example, calcium deficits may be detected by two simple assessments: Trousseau or Chvostek signs.

   — Trousseau's sign is elicited by grasping the person's wrist or inflating a blood pressure cuff to temporarily constrict arterial blood flow. If the fingers flex toward the palm (palmar flexion), the person probably has a serious calcium deficit.

   — Chvostek's sign is elicited by tapping the person's cheek along the facial nerve just below the temple. If the facial muscle twitches, a calcium deficit is probably present.

Diagnostic Testing

Various testing procedures focus on determining the hormone levels or the physiological effect of the hormone.

1. Various laboratory tests are available to determine specific endocrine activities. For example, serum calcium levels reflect parathyroid function. Serum and urine cortisol levels reflect adrenal gland activity.

2. A tracer dose of radioactive iodine is given orally and the thyroid gland is scanned at specified intervals to determine the amount of iodine accumulated in the gland.

3. Several tests are conducted to determine the endocrine function of the pancreas by measuring the response to an intake of glucose. Pre- and post-meal serum glucose levels and urine glucose testing are common procedures that can be monitored by health care providers and learned by the client and family members.

4. A tissue biopsy provides cells to identify infectious or abnormal processes. Cytologic examination of cells may also be performed. The Papanicolaou ("pap") smear obtained by pelvic or gynecological examination identifies the vaginal and cervical cells and fluids.

5. Mammography or thermography are pictorial representations of breast tissue by low-dose radiation or infrared photography to identify nonpalpable or unrecognized lesions.

SECTION 3: CLINICAL EXAMPLES OF COMMON ENDOCRINE CONDITIONS

It is essential to understand the primary function of each gland in order to anticipate an excess or deficit response. It can become very confusing to review both the excess and deficit responses of each gland. It is even more difficult to differentiate the manifestations without having a specific clinical example to refer to. Thus, selected commonly recurring endocrine dysfunction will be presented in this unit. It is suggested to use each example as a point of reference for comparison of similar clinical examples and a point of contrast when opposite hormonal situations occur.

Hyperthyroidism

This clinical syndrome is caused by excess amounts of thyroid hormone in circulation which accentuates all body activity resulting in a hypermetabolic state. Graves' disease (diffuse toxic goiter) is the most common form and can be successfully managed with medication.

1. Clinical manifestations reflecting increased metabolism include increased appetite with weight loss; "wide open" stare appearance of the eyes (exophthalmus); increased vital signs, especially tachycardia and palpitations; increased perspiration with sweaty palms; CNS excitability, anxiety and insomnia. The thyroid is often enlarged (goiter) because of increased stimulation of the gland.

   − Pharmacological management block the synthesis and release of thyroid hormones.

- Antithyroid agents such as propylthiouracil (Propacil, PTU) and methimazole (Tapazole) are taken for long-term management.

- Iodide preparations (potassium iodide, Lugol's solution) are often administered in combination with antithyroid agents.

- Radioactive iodide destroys hyperactive thyroid cells.

- Propranolol (Inderal) is administered to control the cardiac excitability. Barbiturates and tranquilizers are administered to promote rest.

2. Subtotal thyroidectomy may be performed to remove a part of the gland to control hyperactivity or to remove a tumor. As the gland is vascular, post-operative hemorrhage is a possibility. Damage to the laryngeal nerve (hoarseness) and/or to the parathyroid glands (calcium deficiency) are other potential post-operative complications. Edema at the operative site may extend inward and compress the trachea causing a choking sensation and respiratory distress.

   — Manipulation of the gland during surgery may cause a sudden release of thyroid hormone resulting in an acute hypermetabolic state (thyrotoxic crisis or thyroid storm). Tachycardia and elevating body temperature with poor response to antipyretics (acetaminophen/Tylenol) are early indicators of a sudden surge of large amounts of thyroid hormone being released into circulation. This medical emergency is managed in a critical care setting where circulatory consequences are continuously monitored.

3. Inadequate amounts of circulating thyroid hormone leads to progressive decrease in metabolic activity (hypothyroidism). This state may be due to an inadequate intake of iodine, thyroid atrophy, secondary to treatment of hyperthyroidism or withdrawal of thyroid supplemental medications such as synthetic levothyroxine (Synthroid, Cytomel, Thyrolar).

   — With decreased metabolic activity, physiological functions are slowed causing fatigue; weight gain; inability to concentrate; cold intolerance; low vital signs, especially hypotension; thin and dry hair. This decrease in metabolism may progress to a profound state of myxedema coma.

   — Elevated serum cholesterol levels and related atherosclerosis are common. With thyroid replacement therapy, there is an increased risk for angina or myocardial infarction. Therefore, replacement therapy is started in low doses and gradually increased to therapeutic levels.

Hypothyroidism

This condition is typically managed with daily supplementation and is rarely seen as the primary reason for hospitalization. It is a clinical syndrome associated with subnormal levels of thyroid hormone. Symptoms may vary from mild to severe. Failure to take thyroid supplement as treatment of hypothyroidism for an extended period of time may result in a multiple body system failure (myxedema coma).

1. There are four types of hypothyroidism: primary, secondary, goitrous, and transient.

   – Primary hypothyroidism accounts for 90% of cases. The most common cause is atrophy or destruction of thyroid tissue from an autoimmune response.

   – Conditions that affect the pituitary gland or the hypothalamus can result in insufficient stimulation of the thyroid gland. This type of hypothyroidism is called secondary states.

   – Goitrous states are due to defective thyroid hormone synthesis which produces an enlarged gland or goiter. Goitrous disorders include Hasimoto's thyroiditis, iodine deficiency or goitrogenic medications (propylthiouracil, methimazole, lithium or iodine).

   – Transient hypothyroidism may be seen in the immediate postpartum period, in newborns following maternal ingestion of hyperthyroid medication, concurrent with some collagen diseases, or malignancies.

2. Typical clinical manifestations relate to decreased metabolism and cellular functioning. Weakness, fatigue, exercise and cold intolerance are characteristic when seen with very dry skin, alopecia, thinning/absence of lateral eyebrows, weight gain and depressed affect. Symptoms are often minimized when exhibited in persons over 65 years of age.

3. Thyroid function can be successfully restored and maintained with daily oral medication: levothyroxine (Levothroid, Synthroid). For non-transient cases, daily medication is required indefinitely. Cessation of medication will result in the return of hypothyroid state which may progress to multi-system failure.

Hypoparathyroidism

This condition develops when insufficient amounts of parathyroid hormone (PTH) is circulating. It may result from damage or injury during surgical treatment of the thyroid gland. Surgical removal (parathyroidectomy) may be performed to control the adverse effects of prolonged, elevated serum phosphate levels associated with severe end stage renal disease.

1. Serum levels of phosphate and calcium are inversely related and are controlled by parathyroid activity. Therefore, with decreased parathyroid activity (hypoparathyroidism), phosphate levels are elevated and calcium levels are decreased.

   – The body attempts to restore normal calcium by removing calcium from bones (demineralization) leading to osteoporosis.

2. Clinical manifestations of decreased parathyroid function include numbness and tingling around the mouth and fingertips; twitching of skeletal muscles; dysrhythmias; photophobia (eyes are very sensitive to light); positive Chvostek and Trousseau signs.

   – Calcium supplements and Vitamin D are administered to facilitate the gastrointestinal absorption of oral and dietary calcium.

   – Aluminum-containing antacids (Amphogel, Basaljel) bind with phosphorus ions and facilitate their excretion.

Hyperadrenalism (Cushing's Disease)

A combination of symptoms are associated with the prolonged elevation of glucocorticoid (steroids) in circulation. This phenomenon usually is a secondary (iatrogenic) response to the therapeutic administration of steroids for the control of inflammatory or disease process involving other body systems or organs.

1. Clinical manifestation relates to altered metabolism of nutrients and altered inflammatory and immune responses. Symptoms include a characteristic pattern of weight gain (central obesity with large abdomen and thin extremities, fat deposits on the face and neck); thin, transparent skin which bruises easily; generalized osteoporosis; hyperglycemia; increased body hair (hirsutism).

   – Increased blood levels of gluticorticoids activity suppresses the inflammatory reaction. Often only mild symptoms (slight temperature elevation) may be detected even when a serious infection is present.

2. Pharmacological preparation which may lead to this complication include: dexamethasone (Decadron), prednisone, cortisone, triamcinolone (Aristcort), methylprednisolone (Solu-Medrol).

- Suppression of the adrenal cortex may persist up to one year after receiving corticosteroids for only two weeks. Dosages are reduced gradually to allow the return of normal adrenal function. Individuals may remain at risk for adrenal insufficiency in times of stress such as illness or surgery.

- Sudden withdrawal of steroid administration may result in an acute state of hypoadrenalism (Addisonian crisis). As the mobilization of protein and glucose stores are slowed, hypoglycemia develops. There is a loss of vascular tone in the periphery as well as a decreased response to catecholamines, epinephrine and norepinephrine leading to systemic hypotension. Therefore, vascular shock develops rapidly. Sodium is excreted and potassium retained by the kidneys leading to severe systemic electrolyte imbalances and subsequent acute physiological dysfunction. Unless treated rapidly and aggressively, death may occur within hours.

Diabetes Mellitus (DM)

1. Insulin is required for the transport of glucose molecules into cells for normal cellular metabolism. Normally, an increase in blood glucose from ingested food or conversion from stored glycogen stimulates the release of insulin from the Islet (beta) cells in the pancreas. When the pancreas is not able to produce or release sufficient amounts of insulin to maintain blood glucose levels between 60-120 mg/dl, an excess of glucose is in circulation. This state is called diabetes mellitus (DM).

   - Insulin-dependent diabetes mellitus (IDDM) or Type I commonly develops in childhood or early adulthood and accounts for 10% of the cases of diabetes. Individuals with IDDM lack endogenous insulin due to insufficient beta cell function and are totally dependent upon insulin administration for survival.

   - Noninsulin-dependent diabetes mellitus (NIDDM) or Type II is an adult-onset phenomenon. It occurs when metabolic needs or body size exceeds the ability of the pancreas to produce sufficient quantities of insulin for normoglycemia. Individuals with NIDDM may require insulin during times of stress, surgery, infection or when diet and oral hypoglycemic medications fail to control elevated serum glucose levels.

2. DM affects all body systems. Self-management is crucial for maintaining normoglycemia and delaying long-term complications. Due to altered metabolism, blood vessels undergo atherosclerotic changes resulting in cardiovascular consequences. Poorly controlled DM (non-adherence) will lead to the early onset of hypertension, coronary heart disease, cerebral vascular conditions,

renal insufficiency, peripheral vascular insufficiency, neuropathy (sensory impairment), retinopathy (retinal detachment) and impotence.

— Insulin-dependent individuals are at risk for diabetic ketoacidosis (DKA) and hypoglycemia.

— Noninsulin-dependent individuals are at risk for hyperosmolar hyperglycemic nonketonic coma (HHNC) and hypoglycemia.

3. DM is collaboratively managed by the physician, nurse and diabetic individual.

— Dietary intake is planned to achieve an ideal body weight and spaced food ingestion which contains 60% carbohydrate, 20% protein and 20% fat. Through the use of established exchange lists, individuals plan three balanced meals and a bedtime snack to meet individual metabolic needs, activity requirements, and peak action following insulin administration.

— Severe hypoglycemia may develop if a diabetic person receives an unusual dose of insulin and is vomiting, not eating sufficient amounts of food or is NPO.

— Planned, regular exercise is as important as dietary management to maintain normoglycemia and delay the onset of complications. Planned exercise lowers blood glucose levels, maintains normal cholesterol levels and improves circulation. The body's ability to utilize glucose improves.

— Oral hypoglycemic medications (sulfonylureas) are prescribed for NIDDM persons to increase insulin production. Examples of first generation oral hypoglycemic agents include tolbutamide (Orinase), chlorpropamide (Diabinese), and tolazamide (Tolinase). Newer preparations include glyburide (Dio Beta) and glipzide (Glucotrol).

• The most serious side effect is hypoglycemia because these products have a 72-hour duration and half life of an additional 36 hours. Close monitoring for hypoglycemia is required when oral hypoglycemics are administered in combination with other potentially hypoglycemic agents (salicylates, sulfonamides, methyldopa, acetaminophen, haloperidol, marijuana).

• Hypoglycemic preparations are usually discontinued several days before surgery because their long-term effects increase the risk of hypoglycemia. Close monitoring of blood glucose is required and supplemental insulin may be temporally administered by using a sliding scale to adjust dosage to patients' needs.

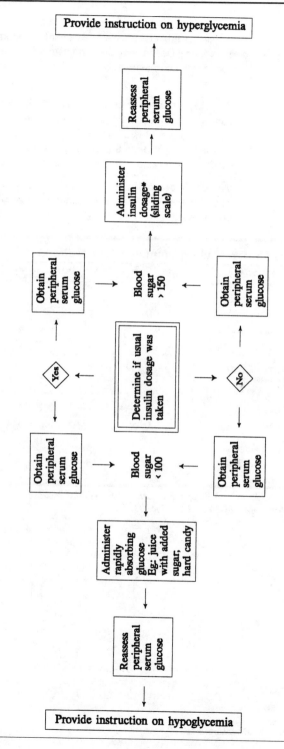

Fig 5-2. Decision Tree for "Flu-like" Symptoms and Insulin - Dependent DM

— Insulin is available as short-, intermediate- and long-acting preparations. Doses may be administered by subcutaneous injection, continuous intravenous infusion (drip) or portable infusion pump.

- Split-dose regimen is currently prescribed as it allows for accurate control over a 24-hour period. Typically 2/3 of the daily requirement is administered in the morning with a smaller dose given in the evening. A combination of intermediate- and rapid-acting insulin preparations is used.

- While all types of insulin can be administered into subcutaneous tissue, only regular insulin can be administered intravenously.

Table 5-1. **Action of insulin preparations**

Type of Insulin	Time of Onset (hr)	Peak of Action (hr)	Duration of Action (hr)	Insulin Appearance
RAPID-ACTING				
Regular	< 1	2-4	4-6	Clear
Crystalline zinc	< 1	2-4	5-8	Clear
Semilente	< 1	4-7	12-16	Cloudy
INTERMEDIATE-ACTING				
NPH	1-2	8-12	18-24	Cloudy
Globin zinc	2-4	6-10	12-18	Clear
Lente	1-4	8-12	18-24	Cloudy
LONG-ACTING				
Protamine zinc	4-8	16-18	36+	Cloudy
Ultralente	4-8	16-18	36+	Cloudy

Adapted from W.J. Phipps, B.C. Long, N.F. Woods: Medical-Surgical Nursing, 5th ed.; St. Louis: Mosby-Year Book, Inc., 1995.

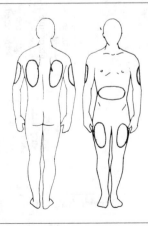

Fig. 5-3. Rotation sites.

Focused Bedside Assessment
(Episode or Onset of DKA)

The following assessment data would be expected with an episode of hyperglycemia (DKA). No other pathophysiological problems involving other body system dysfunction unrelated to DM or DKA are included.

*   **General appearance:** Feels "weak and sleepy;" appears weak and listless; dry, flushed appearance.

*   **Neurological status:** Awakens easily from sleeping periods but slow when responding to questions; blurred vision; headache.

*   **Cardiac status:** Blood pressure lower than baseline; at-rest pulse rate increased (80-90 beats/minute).

*   **Respiratory status:** Breathing deeply and regularly; sweet "fruity" odor to breath; breath sounds clear.

*   **Abdominal (GI) status:** Nausea; possible vomiting and non-localized pain.

*   **Urinary elimination:** Voids frequently in large amounts; urine pale and clear; possible nocturia and incontinence.

*   **Extremities:** Flushed, dry skin.

*   When the individual is turned to their side, the nurse would expect to assess no unusual findings.

If additional data are observed, a more detailed assessment of the involved system is required. Additional areas of physiological dysfunction may be present and confound the present clinical situation of DKA.

---

4. Diabetic Ketoacidosis (DKA)

— This hyperglycemic complication develops when there is a markedly inadequate amount of insulin in circulation. The primary causes are missing doses of insulin or the presence of illness or infection. Physical and emotional stress also increases glucose production.

— Clinical manifestations of an elevated serum glucose level develop over several hours or even days. This clinical situation may develop as a result of: (1) omission of insulin or hypoglycemic medication and eating regularly, (2) prolonged or severe emotional stress; or (3) subtle onset of respiratory, renal or urinary tract infection.

— The elevated osmolality (excess glucose molecules) leads to fluid movement from the interstitial and intracellular spaces into the intravascular compartment. Diuresis of fluid and associated loss of sodium and potassium in the urine may lead to dehydration and electrolyte imbalances.

— When the glucose is unavailable for cellular metabolism, protein and fat stores are utilized. This process is less efficient and results in the accumulation of plasma ketone bodies (ketoacidosis). As the pH lowers, the respiratory center is stimulated producing deep, rapid respirations with a characteristic sweet ("fruity") odor of the breath (Kussmaul respirations). The individual's level of consciousness progressively becomes more lethargic. If untreated the condition leads to coma and possibly death.

- Assessment of serum glucose levels confirms hyperglycemia and ketosis. Depending upon the severity, the condition may be treated in a specialty unit with restoration of electrolyte balance, rehydration and insulin administration. Continuous monitoring of systemic response is required.

5. Hyperosomolar hyperglycemic nonketotic coma (HHNC)

— This hyperglycemic complication develops slowly by individuals who have undiagnosed or inadequately treated non-insulin dependent diabetes mellitus (NIDDM). The degree of hyperglycemia is more profound as compared to DKA; thus, the degree of dehydration is often more severe.

— As acidosis does not develop concurrently with the elevating blood glucose, clinical manifestations are often overlooked. Changes in level of consciousness and lethargy develop later than seen with DKA.

- Treatment is managed in specialty care units as close monitoring of circulatory status is required. Individuals are at risk for altered perfusion complications (renal failure, thromboemboli or cerebral vascular accident).

6. Hypoglycemia (insulin shock)

— A lowering of the blood glucose is usually caused by an overdose of insulin, skipping meals after taking hypoglycemic medication or increased exercise disproportionate to food intake. It develops at the peak action of the hypoglycemic medication or at night when the individual is fasting.

— Clinical manifestations occur when the blood glucose falls rapidly or below 50 mg/dl. Alcohol consumption can also cause hypoglycemia because it depletes glycogen stores.

- Symptoms develop rapidly or progress over a few hours. A progressive headache accompanied by apprehension, double vision and irritability is the typical onset. Slurred speech, trembling, sweating, staggering gait develop quickly. Without prompt treatment, coma and shock develop and a high mortality rate may occur.

Focused Bedside Assessment
(Acute Hypoglycemia/Insulin Shock)

The following assessment data would be expected during an episode of hypoglycemia or insulin shock. No other pathophysiological problems involving other body system dysfunction unrelated to hypoglycemia are presented. This clinical situation may develop as result of: (1) delayed or omission of a meal after taking insulin or hypoglycemic medication; (2) vomiting and/or diarrhea and administration of the same dosage of insulin or hypoglycemic medication; or (3) excessive exercise without adjusting intake.

* **General appearance:** Irritable, restless and nervous; slurred speech; generalized cool, moist skin; pallor; possible diaphoresis.

* **Neurological status:** Headache; visual disturbances; light-headedness; possible confusion or hallucinations; seizures.

* **Cardiac status:** Increased pulse rate; below normal blood pressure; weak, thready pulse rate; palpitations.

* **Respiratory status:** Shallow, increased respiratory rate; possible hyperventilation.

* **Abdominal (GI) status:** Diminished bowel sounds; loss of appetite; numbness of lips and tongue.

* **Urinary elimination:** Diminished output.

* **Extremities:** Cool to cold extremities (possible mottled appearance); diminished peripheral pulses; delayed capillary refill; tremors.

* When the individual is turned to their side, the nurse would expect to assess no unusual findings.

If additional data are observed, a more detailed assessment of the involved system is required. Additional areas of physiological dysfunction may be present and confound an episode of insulin shock.

- Altered consciousness may be misinterpreted as an alcoholic stupor or a response to post-operative analgesia. Check for diaphoresis and moisture of the bedsheets. Sweating is a readily observable sign of insulin shock.

- Prompt administration of a fast-acting carbohydrate will reverse the progression of symptoms. If the individual is conscious, administer 4-6 ounces of fruit juice or nondiet soda; 2 tsp. sugar or honey; 5-7 lifesaver candy or glucose tablets. If the individual is unconscious, IV access is required as 50ml of 50% dextrose is usually prescribed by IV push.

Focused Bedside Assessment
(Long Term DM)

The following assessment data would be expected for an individual who has had adult onset diabetes mellitus (NIDDM) for several years, even when well-controlled, pathophysiological changes associated with secondary atherosclerosis develop. The signs of early onset of these changes and at-risk factors are presented. No other pathophysiological conditions involving other body systems dysfunctions unrelated to DM are presented.

* **General appearance:** Overweight for height and body frame; no acute distress but experiencing general malaise.

* **Neurological status:** Alert; oriented X4; blurring vision; history or chest pain with increased activity (angina); fainting episodes.

* **Cardiac status:** Mild hypertension with elevated diastolic pressure (above 80 mmHg); pulse regular; no abnormal heart sounds.

* **Respiratory status:** Lungs clear; WNL.

* **Abdominal (GI) status:** Abdomen soft; no tenderness; bowel sounds in all quadrants; thirsty.

* **Urinary elimination:** Voids sufficient quantities (qs); some hesitancy and occasional dysuria; nocturia X2; history of recurrent UTI and impotence (in males) or vaginitis (in females).

* **Extremities:** Decreased sensation in toes; both feet pale and cool to touch; pedal pulses present but weaker on one foot; skin intact; no ankle edema; intermittent leg cramping especially with walking or climbing stairs.

* When the individual is turned on their side, the nurse would expect to assess no unusual findings.

If additional data are observed, a more detailed assessment of the involved system is required. Additional areas of physiological dysfunction may be present as secondary atherosclerosis progresses.

- • If consciousness is not promptly regained, more aggressive therapy and continuous monitoring in an intensive care unit is usually warranted.

  - — Sometimes a cycle of rebound hyperglycemia following episodes of hypoglycemia occurs (Somogyi effect). This complication is difficult to manage and usually requires close monitoring of interventions and responses.

7. Long-term complications may develop as a result of changes in the vascular structure. Atherosclerotic changes develop at a younger age in diabetic as compared to non-diabetic individuals. There is a greater risk for coronary artery disease, cerebral vascular accidents, peripheral vascular disease, retinopathy leading to blindness and chronic renal failure.

- Due to the progressive loss of peripheral neural sensation (diabetic neuropathy), diabetics are at risk for soft tissue injury and delayed healing. Individuals may not feel the pain which typically accompanies an infection or tissue injury. Concurrent peripheral vascular insufficiency often leads to skin breakdown, gangrene and amputation of affected parts.

The development of complications increases the cost of health care and decreases the quality of life for poorly controlled diabetic individuals. It is estimated that 50-75% of lower extremity amputations are performed on diabetic individuals. And, 50% of these amputations could have been prevented if daily preventive foot care had been practiced.

SECTION 4: EXAMPLES OF COMMON REPRODUCTIVE CONDITIONS

Conditions Affecting Females

Only those conditions which are most likely to be managed during a hospital stay will be discussed in this section.

1. Pelvic relaxation conditions

    - Conditions resulting in the relaxation of perineal muscles and fascia may lead to displacement of pelvic organs (uterus, urinary bladder and/or the rectum). Factors contributing to the development of structural weakening are aging process, childbirth and pelvic surgery. Pelvic relaxation impairs the physiological functioning of the involved anatomical structures and may interfere with satisfactory sexual intercourse.

    - Cystocele refers to the descent of the urinary bladder and weakened anterior wall of the vagina into the vaginal canal. The protrusion or bulge may interfere with emptying and controlling the urinary bladder, causing loss of urine when a woman sneezes, coughs, laughs or does anything that strains the abdominal muscles.

        • Surgical repair of a cystocele is called an anterior repair or anterior colporrhaphy. Resuming an adequate urinary elimination pattern and complete bladder emptying are essential following this procedure. Due to edema at the operative site, continuous or intermittent catheterization may be required post-operatively or after discharge until sensation and muscle control is restored. Pelvic muscle exercises (Kegel) strengthens perineal and sphincter muscle tone.

— Rectocele refers to the descent of the rectum and weakened posterior wall of the vagina into the vaginal canal. The protrusion or bulge may interfere with defecation causing constipation, a feeling of rectal fullness and incontinence of flatus or feces.

  • Surgical repair of a rectocele is called a posterior repair or posterior colporrhaphy. Adequate fluid intake, increased dietary fiber, stool softeners and regular pattern of elimination facilitate the return of normal bowel habits.

— Uterine prolapse is the descent of the cervix or entire uterus into the vaginal canal due to the relaxation of the ligaments which normally holds the uterus up in the pelvic cavity. While varying degrees of prolapse may occur, it usually does not interfere with the menstrual cycle.

  • Surgical repair of a uterine prolapse is called a uterine suspension and may be combined with repair procedures. Non-surgical intervention involves the use of a removable mechanical device (pessary) which holds the uterus in its normal anatomical position.

2. Tumors

Excessive tissue growth involving the female reproductive organs may be benign or malignant. These conditions usually require some surgical intervention as the primary method of treatment.

— Benign ovarian cysts may occur at any time during the childbearing period as a follicular or corpus luteum cyst depending upon the phase of the menstrual cycle the cyst developed. Most cysts regress spontaneously. If one persists, it may rupture and require surgical intervention.

— Malignant ovarian tumor is the sixth most frequent cancer in women and accounts for more deaths than any other cancer of the female reproductive system. Ovarian cancer has no early symptoms and there are no effective screening techniques to detect it.

— The disease is usually advanced by the time it is diagnosed. It is generally considered a silent disease, meaning that by the time a woman experiences symptoms, the disease usually has spread beyond the primary site.

  • Surgical removal of the tumor, radiation and chemotherapy reduce the tumor size and progression of the disease. The five-year survival has not changed significantly over the past 20 years due to the presence of advanced disease at the time of diagnosis. Five-year survival rates are discouraging.

- Clinical manifestations include pain, abdominal distention or ascites and abnormal vaginal bleeding. Due to mechanical obstruction caused by the tumor size, gastrointestinal symptoms develop (dyspepsia, vomiting, constipation/diarrhea).

- Cervical cancer is another relatively common tumor among women depending upon the age and contributing factors experienced by the woman. It can be diagnosed while it is localized and asymptomatic by the Papanicolaou ("pap") smear. When diagnosed and treated early, the five-year survival rate is favorable. However, some groups of women do not seek regular gynecological examination, and this condition may go undetected. By the time symptoms of abnormal menstrual bleeding accompanied by low back pain are present, the disease has often spread to surrounding tissue.

  - Biopsy and curettage (scraping) of cervical tissue are required to confirm the extent of the cellular involvement.

  - Removal of a cone-shaped segment of the cervix with cautery or laser surgery may be performed for the removal of localized abnormal tissue. These procedures do not affect fertility or childbearing.

  - If the disease has extended wider than cervical tissue, a hysterectomy and bilateral salpingo-oophorectomy ("total hysterectomy") is performed. Radiation with multidrug chemotherapy regimes is used.

- The most common uterine overgrowth involves benign tumors arising from the muscle layer. These growths are called myomas or fibroids. They may occur throughout the uterus but usually are more frequent in the fundus or top of the uterus. They tend to increase in size during pregnancy and with oral contraceptive or estrogen therapy. They are slow growing and therefore can become quite large before becoming symptomatic.

  - Uterine myomas often cause abnormal uterine or menstrual bleeding, pain and symptoms due to pressure on adjacent structures. They rarely progress into a malignancy.

  - A myomectomy refers to the surgical removal of the growth while leaving the uterus intact for women who wish to preserve fertility.

- A hysterectomy is recommended for women who have severe symptoms, have extremely large or multiple growths, and who are past childbearing age. This procedure may be performed through a low abdominal incision, through a vaginal incision or by laproscopic surgical techniques. The approach is dependent upon the size of the uterus, the need for increased visibility of surrounding structures or the need for vaginal repair.

- A total or "pan" hysterectomy includes the removal of the uterus, fallopian tubes and the ovaries. Often, all structures removed are listed: hysterectomy and salpingo-oophorectomy.

- Hormone replacement therapy may be indicated following the removal of ovaries.

— Due to the abundant blood supply to pelvic structures, there is a risk for post-operative bleeding following a hysterectomy. If bleeding occurs from the vaginal incision (where the cervix was removed), there is increased drainage on the perineal pads. Internal bleeding into the abdominal cavity may also occur within the first post-operative hours. Unusually intense abdominal pain, hypotension, tachycardia and a drop in urinary output in spite of an adequate IV fluid intake are warning signs. Drainage from the abdominal incision is rare.

- Menstrual flow ceases following a hysterectomy. Cessation of hormonal supply ceases with the removal of the ovaries (surgical menopause). "Hot flashes", restlessness, insomnia, emotional fluctuations, palpitations or dizziness may develop within 24-48 hours post-operatively. Hormone replacement therapy may be required.

- Refer to Unit 8 for additional discussion on perioperative nursing care.

3. Breast cancer
   Benign disorders of the breast are common among women during the childbearing years. Fibrocystic condition is the most common lesion and usually detected as a painful lump in the breast. Frequently a breast cyst involves the collection of serous fluid within an encapsulated area. Solid benign growths may also develop. All "lumps" should be evaluated. Needle aspiration of the cystic contents is examined in a manner similar to a Papanicolaou evaluation. Incisional biopsy involves the surgical removal of a portion or all of the lump for histologic/cellular evaluation.

   - Differentiating between a benign or malignant condition is done by laboratory examination of the tissue involved. Clinical manifestations are often similar and misleading.

- Surgical biopsy is usually done in ambulatory surgical services or during brief hospitalization. The fear of malignancy is high with the majority of women undergoing this procedure.

— The incidence of breast cancer is second only to lung cancer among women. The type is determined by the tissue origin and influences the course of the disease.

- The first sign of breast cancer is a painless lump which may be similar to a benign fibrocystic growth. Mammography and thermography are used for screening and early detection. A biopsy or lumpectomy provides the definitive diagnosis. Treatment is based upon the extent of the disease process. Surgical removal, radiation and chemo-therapy are utilized.

— Possible surgical procedures

- Lumpectomy is the removal of the tumor mass with or without axillary node removal.

- Subcutaneous mastectomy is the removal of underlying breast tissue leaving the skin, areola and nipple intact.

- Partial mastectomy is the removal of the tumor, surrounding tissue and usually the axillary lymph nodes.

- Simple mastectomy is the removal of the involved breast but not the chest muscles or axillary lymph nodes.

- Modified radical mastectomy is the complete removal of all breast tissue, adjacent soft tissue and axillary nodes.

- Radical mastectomy (Halsted) is the complete removal of the breast, pectoralis major and minor muscles, adjacent fat, fascia and lymph nodes.

— The type of surgery performed determines the extent of post-operative care. A large pressure dressing is usually in place immediately following surgery to minimize fluid collection at the operative site. If dissection under the skin flaps occurred, a closed, negative drainage collection catheter and system are placed (Hemovac, Duval).

— Radiation is used for inflammatory carcinoma and advocated by some physicians following a lumpectomy.

— Chemotherapy (adjuvant) is advocated by some physicians following a lumpectomy and for women with recurrence, metastasis, or high risk for recurrence. An indwelling catheter (Hickman, Broviac, Groshong) or implantable infusion port

(Porta-cath) may be inserted at the time of surgery. Refer to Unit 8 for additional discussion about oncological nursing care.

- The excised tissue is analyzed to determine the hormone receptor (estrogen or progesterone). Hormone-dependent malignant tumors determine the potential benefit of endocrine chemotherapy or removal of the ovaries to retard the recurrent growth and spread of the tumor.

— Due to incisional pain, edema and retraction of operated tissue, movement of the affected arm is often diminished. Encouragement to participate in personal hygiene is the initial focus of exercise and activity. Progressive activities are planned to systematically increase the range of movement to ensure maximum shoulder flexion and rotation. With the consent of the physician, "Reach for Recovery" volunteers from the American Cancer Society are beneficial.

— With the removal of lymph nodes, there is a risk of impaired lymphatic drainage. Giving injections, drawing blood specimens and taking blood pressures on the affected arm are avoided; thus, minimizing tissue injury and possible delayed healing.

- Keeping the arm elevated to the level of the heart minimizes fluid accumulation in the affected arm. Care focuses on maintaining skin integrity and minimizing the possibility of infection.

— Temporary prostheses are available in various contours, consistency and weights to augment or replace removed tissue. Reconstructive surgery is delayed until the course of treatment is completed and the risk of recurrence is low.

Conditions Affecting Males

1. Priapism refers to the prolonged penile erection that is painful and is not associated with sexual arousal. It may occur to males with spinal cord trauma, sickle cell crisis, acute, undiagnosed leukemia or pelvic tumors. The vascular spaces of the penis remain engorged leading to thrombosis and secondary edema of surrounding tissue. Conservative treatment initiated within hours of onset is effective and prevents impotence. Interventions may include iced saline enemas, spinal anesthesia, or needle aspiration of the collected blood with pressure dressings.

2. Testicular cancer

   — Malignancy of the testes is relatively rare among all men but is
   the most common malignancy among young males 25-35
   years of age. Usually one testis is involved. Testicular enlargement or irregularity is an early sign detected by self examination. Surgical removal (orchiectomy) with radiation and/or
   chemotherapy is recommended. Refer to Unit 8 for additional
   discussion on oncological nursing care.

3. Prostatic enlargement

   — Benign prostatic hypertrophy (BPH) is a common condition
   which occurs with increasing frequency as males become
   older. It is estimated that approximately half of all men over
   the age of 65 have some prostatic enlargement. As the prostate gland enlarges slowly, the urinary urethra is progressively
   compressed causing symptoms of urinary retention and status-
   induced infection. As the treatment focuses on restoring and
   maintaining adequate urinary drainage, the specific interventions are discussed in Unit 6.

     • Elderly men may be treated for one physiological problem
       and concurrently have varying degrees of BPH. The re-
       sponse to interventions, changes in diet/fluid intake, or medi-
       cations for a current condition may also impact on urinary
       function and exaggerate the symptoms associated with
       BPH. Therefore, it is essential to establish the "normal" or
       usual urinary elimination patterns of elderly men at hospital
       admission and prior to the initiation of interventions.
       Changes in an individual's pattern may indicate early signs
       of a developing complication.

     • Nocturia frequently occurs with BPH. The unfamiliar setting
       of the hospital and the use of siderails may lead to falling in-
       juries during the night. The use of night lights, call signals,
       the convenient placement of the urinal and frequent assess-
       ments of the individuals provide opportunities for assisting
       the elderly male patient to the bathroom; thus, minimizing
       falling accidents.

   — Prostatic cancer is a common type of cancer in men over the
   age of 50 years. The initial symptoms mimic the symptoms of
   BPH. Typically this malignant growth progresses slowly but
   does metastasize to surrounding tissue, hips or the lumbar vertebrae.

     • It is recommended that men over age 50 have an annual
       rectal exam of the prostate gland, a serum alkaline phos-
       phatase and serum radioimmunoassay of prostatic acid

phosphatase. These tests detect the condition before clinical symptoms appear.

- Complete surgical removal of the prostate gland (radical prostatectomy), vas deferens and seminal vesicles is recommended through a perineal or retropubic approach. Chemotherapy and/or radiation is recommended if the growth has spread beyond the gland. As this tumor is androgen (testosterone) supported, an orchiectomy (removal of the testes) and/or estrogen therapy may be recommended if recurrence develops.

4. Secondary infections from the male urinary tract
   - The presence of concurrent physiological conditions and interventions may aggravate a minor urinary problem for many adult males. For example, elderly men often have a subacute, asymptomatic urinary tract infection which is secondary to an enlarged prostate gland. This infection may become accentuated during periods of inactivity or altered fluid intake. Due to the close proximity of anatomical structures and the connecting duct system, microorganisms can readily travel along the reproductive ducts leading to secondary infections. These conditions usually respond to antibiotic therapy.

     - Prostatitis is the inflammation or infection of the prostate gland. If this condition is limited to the gland, symptoms include low back pain and perineal pain. The inflammatory edema often obstructs the urethra, causing increased urinary urgency, frequency and nocturia. If there is an associated urinary bladder infection, dysuria, hematuria or cloudy urine is observed.

     - Epididymitis is an inflammation or infection of the epididymis often caused by reflux or "back flow" from the urethra through the vas deferens. Acute onset is associated with painful scrotal swelling and fever.

     - Orchitis is an acute testicular inflammation or infection. The testes become edematous and extremely tender with reddened scrotum. A fever is usually present which indicates systemic involvement. If fluid collects along the spermatic cord, the condition is called a hydrocele. Antibiotics, bedrest with scrotal support and analgesics control the infectious process and minimize the possibility of altered sperm count and sterility.

unit *6*

NURSING CARE OF ADULTS WITH

Urinary Elimination
Conditions

T*his unit addresses common recurring conditions of adults which affect the formation and elimination of urine. The care of individuals with urinary elimination dysfunction on general medical-surgical nursing units is addressed. The management and care of critical and unstable conditions which require continuous monitoring are not addressed in this unit. Examples of clinical conditions requiring high acuity care include: acute renal failure, care during hemodialysis, renal transplantation and continuous arteriovenous hemofiltration.*

SECTION 1: OVERVIEW

Effective plans for care are based upon an understanding of the normal functioning of the renal system. The kidneys are major filtering systems which connect with the urinary tract. The structures for urine elimination include ureters, urinary bladder, urethra and meatus. In males, the prostate gland which surrounds the urethra at the base of the urinary bladder is closely associated with effective and efficient urinary elimination.

Adequate renal function is interrelated with other body system functioning. For example, dysfunction of the heart and decreased pumping capacity directly affects the filtration capacity of the kidneys. In a similar comparison, if renal dysfunction leads to inadequate fluid or electrolyte elimination, fluid retention, hypertension and peripheral edema occurs.

Anatomical Considerations Involving Renal System

The renal system is comprised of the two kidneys and the structures for urinary elimination.

1. The kidneys are located posterior to the abdominal wall and outside the peritoneal cavity. They lie on each side of the vertebral column between the twelfth thoracic and third lumbar vertebrae. The kidneys are protected by a firm capsule and a layer of fatty tissue.

2. The outer surface (cortex) of the kidney is comprised of glomeruli where filtration from the blood occurs. The inner component (medulla) contains the tiny tubular network where appropriate amounts of fluid and substances are reabsorbed back into the circulation. The center portion (renal pelvis) collects the fluid and substances (urine) which remain after reabsorption before it drains into the urinary elimination tract.

3. The nephron is the working unit of the kidney. There are 1.2 million nephrons in each adult kidney. Each nephron includes the major filtrating component (glomerulus) and a tubular network (proximal, Loop of Henle, convoluted and distal tubules). Bowman's capsule is a tiny ball-like structure which includes the glomerulus and the renal arterioles. The wall of the arterioles and the adjacent epithelium of the glomerulus form a semi-permeable membrane. Fluid, nutrients and electrolytes move across the membrane or are filtered from the blood into the renal structures. Various physiological factors and pressure differences determine the amount of filtrate formed.

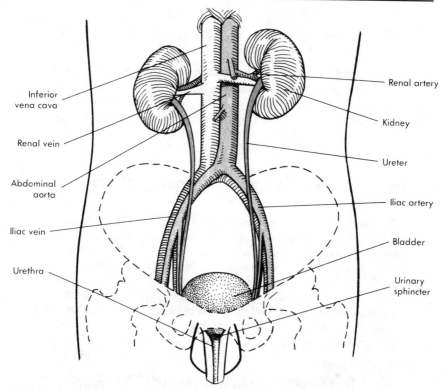

Fig. 6-1. Organs and structures of urinary system. From W.J. Phipps, B.C. Long, N.F. Woods: Medical-Surgical Nursing: Concepts and Clinical Practices, 5th ed.; St. Louis: Mosby-Year Book, Inc., 1995. Reprinted with permission.

Labels on figure: Inferior vena cava, Renal vein, Abdominal aorta, Iliac vein, Urethra, Renal artery, Kidney, Ureter, Iliac artery, Bladder, Urinary sphincter

4. The blood flow continues beyond the glomeruli to the area of the tubules. Arterioles surround the tubules to permit reabsorption of selected amounts of fluid, nutrients and electrolytes back into the circulation. Various physiological factors determine the degree of reabsorption.

5. The fluid, nutrients and electrolytes not reabsorbed form the urine which flows along the tubules and drain into the central collecting area within each kidney (renal pelvis). The first portion of the urine elimination tract are the ureters which connect the renal pelvis to the urinary bladder which is located midline behind the pubic bone. This storage structure can increase in size to hold large amounts of urine. Contraction of the bladder (urination, voiding or micturition) results in urine flow into the urethra and is eliminated through the urinary meatus. Sphincter muscles are located at the exit opening of the bladder and at the meatus for voluntary and involuntary control of elimination.

— The female urethra is approximately 4 cm in length, whereas, in males it is 20 cm in length.

6. In males, the prostate gland surrounds the urethra at the base of the bladder. At this point secretions from the male reproductive system enter the urinary tract. The gland is surrounded by a firm capsule. Therefore as it enlarges with the aging process, it compresses or constricts the urethral opening.

Normal Physiological Functioning of the Renal System

The primary function of the kidneys is to maintain a stable internal environment for optimal cell and tissue activity. The kidneys accomplish this function by regulating fluid, nutrients and electrolytes which circulate in the blood. The desired balance between acid and base ions within our bodies is also regulated by renal activity. Its endocrine functions include the secretion of selected hormones to regulate blood pressure, red blood cell production and calcium metabolism. The end result of renal activities is in the formation of urine which is excreted through a series of tube-like structures.

1. Fluid regulation
   — The kidneys are very vascular receiving 1000-1200 ml of blood/minute or 20-25% of the blood pumped from the heart with each heart beat (cardiac output). The amount of blood passing through the renal circulation is called renal blood flow (RBF) or 600 ml/minute. Various physiological factors within the renal arteries or general circulation affect the adequacy of blood supply (renal perfusion).

   — The amount of fluid and substances that passes from the renal arterioles across the semi-permeable membrane in the glomerulus is called the glomerular filtration rate (GFR). It normally is 125 ml/minute or 7.5 Liters/hour. This filtrate flows from the glomerulus into the network of tubules where fluid, selected nutrients and electrolytes are selectively reabsorbed and returned to the circulation. Various physiological factors or medications affect the degree of reabsorption.

     • Normally, 99% of the filtrate is reabsorbed back into the circulation. Only a few milliliters or 1% remain after reabsorption and pass into the elimination structures. The elimination of urine is also called excretion, voiding, urination or micturition.

     • Normal volume of urine excreted daily is 1-2 Liters or 1000-2000 ml. Minimally adequate hourly output is 30 ml. Ap-

proximately 200-300 ml in the bladder produces the sensation or urge to urinate.

— The renal arterioles contract and relax to maintain fairly constant renal blood flow, filtration and reabsorption rates. This
process of autoregulation is achieved with arterial blood pressures between 80 and 180 mmHg. Without this protective
mechanism a person would be depleted of fluid and electrolytes in less than 5 minutes.

— The renal arteries are also influenced by sympathetic neural
impulses that cause vasoconstriction. For example, when the
general arterial blood pressure falls below 80 mmHg, the renal
arterioles constrict and the renal blood flow (RBF) decreases.
As a result, there is a decrease in filtration and an increase in
reabsorption to ensure an adequate fluid volume within the
vascular system. Physical exercise, body position and hypoxia stimulate a similar response.

— Vasoconstriction, filtration and reabsorption are also influenced
by hormonal responses. The renin-angiotensin cycle is triggered in response to a decrease in renal blood flow. Renin is
released in the glomerulus and forms angiotensin I. It converts to angiotensin II in the lungs resulting in generalized vasoconstriction to increase or maintain an adequate arterial
blood pressure. Angiotensin II converts to Angiotensin III in
the adrenal glands which stimulate the release of aldosterone.
The renal arteries and tubules respond to increased levels of
circulating aldosterone by increasing the reabsorption of sodium. In turn increased amounts of fluid are also reabsorbed.
The end result is retention of fluid within the vascular system
to increase or maintain generalized arterial blood pressure.

2. Electrolyte regulation

   — Electrolytes are small molecules and readily pass into the glomerulus and move back into circulation. Coordinated balance
   between selected filtration and tubular reabsorption, maintains
   serum electrolyte levels within normal parameters. For example, 99.5% of the filtered sodium and 94% of the filtered potassium are reabsorbed.

   — Glucose molecules move freely across the glomerular membrane and are readily reabsorbed. When serum glucose levels are greater than 180 mg/dl, the excess is excreted in the
   urine. (Normal, non-diabetic, serum glucose parameter: 60-
   120mg/dl.)

     • Because the glucose molecule also attracts the water mole-
     cule, there is decreased water reabsorption and increased
     urine formation (polyuria) associated with elevated serum

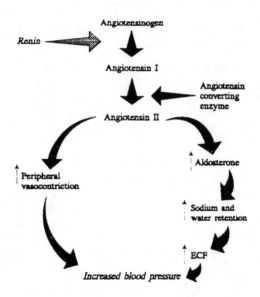

Fig. 6-2. Renin-angiotensin cycle. Adapted from S.M. Lewis, I.C. Collier: Medical-Surgical Nursing: Assessment and Management of Clinical Problems, 4th ed.; St. Louis: Mosby-Year Book, Inc., 1995.

and urine glucose levels. Without adequate fluid intake, dehydration develops.

3. Excretion of metabolic waste products

— Urea is one end-product of protein metabolism. The glomerulus freely filters urea from the blood. As this substance is toxic to other body tissues, especially the brain, it is essential that excess amounts are excreted in the urine.

• The presence of urea in the renal filtrate has a secondary positive effect. It contributes to the kidney's ability to concentrate urine by increasing fluid reabsorption. Therefore, individuals in catabolic, protein depleted or cachexic states are at risk for inadequate urine concentration leading to dehydration.

— Creatinine is another end product of cellular metabolism and muscle breakdown. It is normally produced at a fixed and uniform rate throughout the day. It is not influenced by dietary intake. Therefore, it is a good indicator of the filtration ability of the kidneys.

— The membrane of the glomerulus is relatively impervious to large cells and substances. Blood cells and plasma proteins normally do not pass into the renal filtrating and collecting structures and therefore are not present in the urine. The presence of these larger cells in the urine increases the urinary specific gravity.

— Medications are directly excreted by the kidneys or are metabolized in the liver into inactive forms which are then excreted by the kidneys. Because of this role, some medications cause damage to renal tissue (nephrotoxic). Astute observation for the onset of side and toxic effects may warrant dosage adjustments.

4. Acid-base regulation

— Metabolic processes in the body generally produce acids (carbon dioxide, pyruvic and lactic acids). The respiratory and renal systems achieve balanced acid-base state (homeostasis).

— The filtration and reabsorption capability of the kidneys regulates the balance between the hydrogen ions (acid) and the bicarbonate ions (base) to maintain a plasma/serum pH between 7.35-7.45. When the serum is acidic (pH < 7.35), bicarbonate ions are reabsorbed back into circulation and hydrogen ions are excreted in the urine. When the serum is alkaline (pH > 7.45), hydrogen ions are reabsorbed back into circulation and bicarbonate ions are excreted in the urine. In addition, kidneys have the capability of generating bicarbonate ions from available hydrogen, carbon dioxide.

5. Erythropoiesis

— Erythropoietin is a hormone released by the kidneys in response to a decreased oxygen level in the blood (hypoxia) delivered to the kidneys. Erythropoietin stimulates the bone marrow to produce more red blood cells and prolongs the life of existing RBCs.

6. Regulation of phosphate and calcium

— Vitamin D is converted to its active form by the kidneys. Vitamin D is necessary for absorption of calcium from the gastrointestinal tract and to promote deposition of calcium within the bone.

Variations Related to Aging

1. With aging, there is a gradual decrease in renal blood flow and glomerular filtration rate. The number of nephrons also decreases. It is estimated that the number of functioning nephrons decreases by 30-50% which affects an elder's capacity to compensate for changes in other body system functioning.

   — Decreased numbers of functioning nephrons delays the elimination of medications in the urine. An accumulation of medications in the plasma may lead to toxic effects.

2. Glucose and bicarbonate ions are not as efficiently reabsorbed with advancing age. Sudden changes in the serum pH and circulating fluids may lead to serious imbalances. Fluid loss due to diarrhea or vomiting may precipitate renal insufficiency in an elderly person.

   — Glucose filtration and reabsorption are altered among the elderly resulting in slightly elevated parameters: 52-135 mg/dl.

3. The renin-angiotensin cycle becomes less responsive to systemic changes. The ability to conserve sodium and excrete potassium is decreased. There also is a decreased ability to conserve water and concentrate the urine. Thus, the ability to adjust to intravascular changes is significantly decreased.

4. The aging effects on the reproductive system have secondary effects on urinary elimination.

   — In females, pelvic relaxation may lead to protrusion of the urinary bladder into the vaginal canal. This condition may lead to urinary retention and increases the possibility of cystitis (infection of the urinary bladder) which may ascend into the kidneys. Relaxation of sphincter control may lead to decreased elimination control and stress incontinence. Simple activities, such as sneezing or coughing, often causes spontaneous urinary elimination of a few drops to complete bladder emptying.

   — In males, the prostate gland which surrounds the urethra just below the urinary bladder progressively enlarges constricting the urethral opening. Difficult urination with retention of urine in the bladder lead to recurrent urinary bladder infections. The possibility of microorganisms ascending the urinary tract may lead to kidney and systemic infections.

SECTION 2: RENAL DYSFUNCTION

Overview

Renal and urinary function can be affected by a variety of changes in physiological functioning and disease processes. Because the kidneys filters the blood, renal dysfunction directly impacts on the functioning of other organ systems. In a converse manner, dysfunction of another body system affects the adequacy of renal function and the viability of renal tissue.

Persons with an acute unstable renal problem are usually admitted to specialty units where major body system function is closely monitored. However, at-risk persons may be admitted to a general medical-surgical nursing unit for a non-renal problem. These individuals may also have asymptomatic or marginal renal function which permits adequate elimination of waste products in most situations. Relatively minor deviations in health and circulatory status may disrupt the adequacy and precipitate acute renal insufficiency/failure. It is important for the non-critical care nurse to recognize at-risk persons and situations that may alter the individual's renal function. Under most circumstances these situations can be modified. The severity of renal dysfunction and the development of complications can be averted.

The following examples are common clinical situations that may disrupt renal homeostasis and may lead to an acute renal episode and damage to renal tissue:

* Repeated administration of nephrotoxic medications in high doses (aminoglycides; tetracyclines, anti-neoplastic agents, amphotericin B)

* An elderly person with poorly controlled diabetes mellitus and/or malignant hypertension

* Presence of clinical situations which may impair the perfusion to the kidneys (decreased cardiac output, beta hemolytic streptococcal infections, systemic shock)

Renal insufficiency refers to the decline to about 25% of normal kidney functioning. Seventy-five percent of a kidney cannot effectively filter waste products and control fluid balance. However, if one kidney is impaired, the other kidney will compensate and the overall filtering capability is adequate. Therefore, the degree of damage may not be detected unless both kidneys are impaired.

Renal failure refers to a more significant loss with less than 10% of renal function remaining. Renal failure, acute or chronic, can be a life-threatening condition.

Assessment of Renal/Kidney Status

1. Fluid status

   — As intake and output (I&O) normally are balanced, an imbalance warrants further evaluation. When fluid intake exceeds urine production or urinary output, renal dysfunction may be present.

   — Accurate calculation of fluid intake and output is required when renal dysfunction is suspected. Day-to-day calculations ("running I&O") which detect on-going excesses or deficits are helpful in identifying trends suggestive of subtle dysfunction. Daily body weight is a good indicator of fluid gains or losses. An increase of 2.2 pounds or 1 Kilogram in body weight is equivalent to 1000 ml of retained fluid.

   — Urinary specific gravity is a noninvasive test of the kidneys' ability to concentrate urine and the permeability of the glomerulus. When large cells are present in the urine, the specific gravity is increased which is associated with increased glomerular filtration rather than the ability to concentrate urine.

     • Low urine specific gravity (<1.010) suggests dilute urine. A high urine specific gravity (>1.020) suggests concentrated urine or the pressence of large cells in the urine (protein, bacteria, WBC or RBC)

     • A fixed or unchanging specific gravity inspite of varying fluid intake suggests renal damage.

2. Urine appearance

   — Identifying baseline data about an individual's normal pattern of urinary elimination is helpful when changes are anticipated. Normally urine varies between pale straw-colored to deep yellow. Some foods and medications alter the color and odor of urine.

     • Dysuria refers to pain or burning with the passing of urine.

     • Frequency refers to voiding at more frequent intervals with smaller or larger amounts.

     • Urgency refers to the need to void immediately.

     • Nocturia refers to awakening at night with the need to void.

     • Hesitancy refers to difficulty initiating voiding which is often accompanied by a decrease in force or flow of the urinary stream.

     • Urinary incontinence refers to the lack of voluntary control of voiding.

- Polyuria refers to increased volume of urine produced, usually in amounts greater than 2500 ml/day.

- Oliguria refers to decreased volume of urine produced, usually less than 400 ml/day. This symptom is differentiated from retention of urine in the bladder or other structures.

- Anuria refers to a decrease in urinary production less than 100 ml/day or the cessation of urine production. This symptom is associated with the retention of electrolytes and altered acid-base state characteristic of renal failure.

3. Characteristics of the urine

   - When red blood cells are present in the urine, it appears pink-tinged to bright red in color. This symptom (hematuria) is often accompanied by dysuria, frequency and urgency.

   - When the urine appears cloudy, phosphate salts, bacteria, nitrates or vaginal secretions may be present in the urine. This symptom is often accompanied by dysuria, frequency and urgency.

   - Other large cells are not normally found in the urine: WBC, proteins and ketone bodies. The presence of these substances may be related to increased glomerular permeability and renal damage.

Interpretation of Arterial Blood Gases (ABG)

The human body functions best in a state of homeostasis or balance. Sometimes physiological dysfunction disrupts this balance which may be reflected in an alteration in the acid-base balance. Considerable data gained from an ABG or a series of values increase the understanding of appropriate nursing action and medical management of individual clients.

The changes in acid-base balance discussed in this unit are related to an underlying metabolic or renal condition. The kidneys are marvelous regulators for maintaining and restoring homeostasis. When they are unable to achieve this balance, a metabolic acid-base imbalance occurs which is reflected in changes in the bicarbonate (HCO_3) value. The body's mechanism to restore balance by the pulmonary system is referred to as respiratory compensation.

When interpreting a given ABG, these steps are followed:

1. First look at the pH.

   - Normal parameters (WNL) for serum pH are: 7.35-7.45.

— If the pH of a given ABG is below 7.35, the acid-base imbalance is acidosis.

— If the pH of a given ABG is above 7.45, the acid-base imbalance is alkalosis.

2. The second step determines the type of acid-base imbalance. Look at the $paCO_2$ and HCO_3 values. At this time only those ABG values associated with an underlying metabolic condition are presented.

    — Normal parameters (WNL) for HCO_3 are: 22-26 mEq/L.

    — If the HCO_3 value is below 22 mEq/L. and the pH is below 7.35, then the primary acid-base imbalance is metabolic acidosis.

    — If the HCO_3 value is above 26 mEq/L, and the pH is above 7.45, then the primary acid-base imbalance is metabolic alkalosis.

    — With an elevated HCO_3 value and a $paCO_2$ value WNL, the acid- base imbalance is called UNCOMPENSATED metabolic alkalosis. With a below-normal HCO_3 value and a $paCO_2$ value WNL, the acid-base imbalance is called UNCOMPEN-SATED metabolic acidosis. These responses are not likely to occur because normal lungs and respiratory activity will respond within a few minutes to a metabolic problem.

    — If the HCO_3 value is WNL and the $paCO_2$ value is above or below normal parameters (34-45 mmHg), then a respiratory imbalance is present which is discussed in Unit 2: Nursing Care of Adults with Respiratory (Pulmonary) Conditions.

3. The third step: Identify if compensation by the respiratory system is present and to what extent. The $paCO_2$ value provides an indication of the respiratory system's ability to balance the metabolic acid-base imbalance. Normal respiratory function is able to increase or decrease the depth and rate of breathing in an attempt to exhale or retain carbon dioxide which acts as an acid. The pH value will reflect the effectiveness of compensation to restore homeostasis.

    — Normal parameters for $paCO_2$ are: 35-45 mmHg.

    — When metabolic acidosis is present (HCO_3 < 22 mEq/L), respiratory compensation will be reflected by gradual lowering in the $paCO_2$ value below the normal parameter (<35 mmHg). Remember that the carbon dioxide acts like an acid when in the blood. Thus, when the carbon dioxide level is below nor-

— mal, respiratory alkalosis is present. As this occurs, the pH
will rise toward normal (7.35) but will not be WNL.

— When metabolic alkalosis is present (HCO_3 > 26 mEq/L.), respiratory compensation will be reflected by a gradual rise in
the $paCO_2$ value above the normal parameter (> 45 mmHg).
The pH will decrease toward normal (7.45) but is not WNL.
These acid-base imbalances are called <u>COMPENSATING</u> metabolic acidosis or alkalosis.

— When the respiratory compensation balances the metabolic imbalance, the pH will be WNL. A balance between a primary
metabolic acid-base imbalance and respiratory compensation
is called <u>COMPENSATED</u> metabolic acidosis or alkalosis.

Diagnostic Testing of Renal Status

1. Urination and urinalysis

   Deviations from normal parameters or changes from an
   individual's baseline warrants further assessment.

   — Protein, RBC, WBC and bacteria are not normally found in the
   urine. A few of these cells may be present in a clean catch or
   voided specimen.

   — When fluid intake exceeds urinary output, fluid is retained
   within the vascular compartment which contributes to systemic
   hypertension. Excess fluid may also move into the interstitial
   space and be detected as weight gain or dependent edema.

2. Bladder function

   — Direct visualization

     • Cystoscopy is the direct visualization of the bladder through
     a lighted tube.

     • Cystogram and cystometrogram are procedures involving
     the instillation of dye or fluid into the bladder for visualiza-
     tion and/or measurement of bladder tone.

3. Renal function

   — X-ray

     • A KUB (kidneys, ureters and bladder) involves a flat plate x-
     ray of the abdomen and pelvis. No special preparation is
     necessary.

   An IVP (intravenous pyelography) is the x-ray visualization of the
   urinary tract after the IV injection of a radiopaque dye. Sensitivity
   to the iodine dye may produce an allergic reaction.

— Scans following the injection of radioactive isotopes, ultrasound and CT scans are additional procedures for determining
renal pathology.

— Electrolyte levels are indicators of renal filtration and reabsorption capability especially when evaluated in association with
other abnormalities.

  • Potassium is found in most foods and liquids and is the
    major element within the cells. In order to maintain the nor-
    mal parameters in the serum for optimal cellular activity,
    daily excretion of potassium must equal dietary intake and
    other sources of potassium. With renal damage, serum po-
    tassium levels increase greater than 5.0 mEq/L.

  • One of the major ways the body maintains acid-base bal-
    ance is selective retention or excretion of hydrogen (acid)
    and bicarbonate (base) ions. In addition, normal kidneys
    are capable of generating bicarbonate ions. With renal dys-
    function, metabolic acidosis develops. On an ABG, the
    HCO_3 value decreases below 24 mEq/L.

— Blood Urea Nitrogen (BUN) is a serum test to determine the
kidney's ability to excrete the nitrogenous waste products of
protein metabolism or tissue breakdown. With kidney and/or
liver dysfunction, the BUN value increases above 20
mg/100ml.

  • The ratio between a BUN and creatinine value is a more de-
    finitive assessment of renal dysfunction. Normal parameter
    is 20:1.

— An elevation in serum creatinine values above 1.2 mg/dl is a
reliable indicator of renal dysfunction. Creatinine clearance is
more diagnostic for elderly persons as their serum creatinine
is often WNL despite renal dysfunction.

— Due to diminished erythropoietic ability associated with renal
dysfunction, the red blood cell (RBC) count decreases and the
hematocrit (Hct) falls.

Measures to Improve Renal Functioning

1. Provide adequate fluid intake to ensure adequate urine production
    and urinary output. An estimate of fluid intake is based upon
    body weight. For the first 10 Kg of BW, 100ml/Kg or 1000ml. For
    11-20 Kg of BW, 50 ml/Kg or 500ml. For additional Kg of BW,
    20ml/Kg. Example: for a person weighing 72 Kg, 1000ml (1-10
    Kg @ 100ml/Kg), 500ml (11-20Kg @ 50ml/Kg) and 1040ml (21-
    72Kg @ 20ml/Kg) for a 24-hour fluid intake of 2540 ml.

- If the person is experiencing excess fluid loss from diaphoresis, vomiting or diarrhea, then the fluid intake is adjusted to include the estimated loss.

- When the urinary output is disproportionately less than the fluid intake, the bedside nurse is alert for possible renal dysfunction. When the urinary output decreases to less than 50ml/hour, assessment for the cause is initiated. An hourly output below 30ml, warrants prompt notification of the physician for corrective interventions for the restoration of an adequate output.

- Increased oral fluid intake is one corrective intervention if the underlying physiological condition permits. When a bolus of 300 cc of IV fluid is prescribed, a prompt increase in urine output results when renal function is adequate.

2. If increased urinary output is not achieved by a fluid bolus, then a diuretic may be prescribed. This group of agents selectively blocks the reabsorption of sodium and water from the renal tubules with a resultant increase in urinary output. It should be remembered that with a sudden elimination of urine there is a comparable decrease in intravascular fluid. Orthostatic hypotension with an increased risk for falling may occur, especially for an elderly person.

   - Electrolytes may be excreted along with the fluid, especially potassium and sodium. Assessment for clinical manifestations and laboratory values are indicated to prevent secondary (iatrogenic) complications.

3. As sodium attracts water, the reduction of sodium intake is another approach to control fluid retention. Reducing dietary salt seasoning is difficult for some persons. However, dietary intake of sodium usually far exceeds the requirements for cellular function. Diet history reveals sources of excess sodium intake. Severely restricted sodium diets are usually not well adhered to by patients; therefore, "no-added" salt dietary instructions are more likely to be followed.

4. When the kidneys fail to provide balanced fluid intake/output and to remove the end products of cellular metabolism, life threatening consequences develop. The accumulation of potassium poses a crisis situation as lethal cardiac dysrhythmias may occur. In most situations, the following interventions are performed in critical care settings where continuous cardiac monitoring is available. However, the intervention may be initiated on a medical-surgical nursing unit.

— Prevention of the accumulation of excess potassium in circulation (hyperkalemia) is essential as the risk for lethal ventricular dysrhythmias increases. Initial prevention focuses on dietary restrictions limiting the intake to only meeting daily requirements.

   • Elevated serum levels may be temporarily lowered by the intravenous administration of hypertonic glucose and insulin which moves the excess potassium ions from the serum into the cells.

   • Intravenous calcium counteracts the effects that excess potassium has on the heart muscle, thereby minimizing the risk of ventricular dysrhythmias.

   • Kayexalate (sodium polystyrene sulfonate) is administered orally or rectally. This ion exchange resin attracts and binds with potassium in the large intestine and is then excreted. Depending upon the extent of use, diarrhea often occurs.

   • Dialysis is the most effective treatment and is required for on-going management of elevated serum potassium levels.

5. Restoration of urine flow
   — As the renal pelvis only holds 5 ml, the prompt initiation of measures to restore urine flow is essential to prevent renal damage when urine flow is obstructed.

   — Catheterization is the placement of a sterile tube at several places along the urinary tract to facilitate drainage. Flow by gravity is a natural process, therefore the collecting bag should always be kept below the level of the bladder. The longer a catheter is used, the greater the risk for acquiring an infection.

   • Catheters may be placed through the urethra into the bladder, through the abdominal wall into the bladder (suprapubic approach) or into the ureter or pelvis of the kidney (nephrostomy tube).

   • An indwelling catheter is secured to the body to minimize an in-and-out movement or tension within the bladder. Catheter alignment should approximate the normal anatomical position of the urethra. For women, the catheter is secured along the inner aspect of the thigh. For men, the catheter is secured onto the lower abdomen to straighten the penoscrotal angle and minimize trauma.

If urinary output is not restored CONTACT PHYSICIAN document findings and actions.

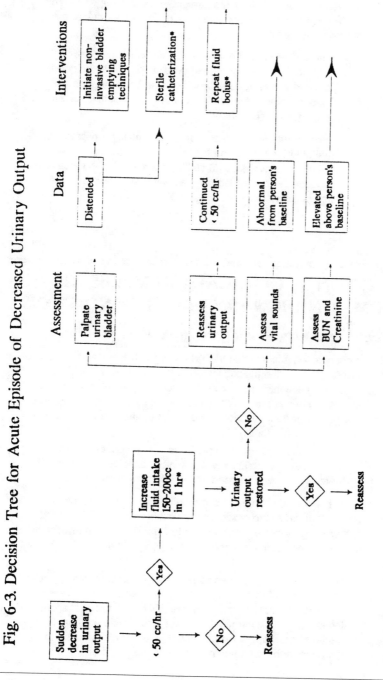

Fig 6-3. Decision Tree for Acute Episode of Decreased Urinary Output

* As prescribed

— For bladder atony, an intermittent catheterization program is
an alternative to long-term indwelling catheterization. The procedure includes inserting a straight urethral catheter into the
bladder at specified time intervals, draining the urine and removing the catheter.

- The catheter may be inserted by the individual (self-catheterization) or another trained person. Sterile technique is
followed in health care facilities because of the high risk of
nosocomial infections. While in the home setting, clean
technique is recommended.

- Intermittent bladder distention and emptying replicates normal bladder function and reactivates the bladder's normal
antibacterial activities. It also increases independence and
reduces the complications associated with long-term retention catheterization.

SECTION 3: CLINICAL EXAMPLES OF COMMON URINARY TRACT CONDITIONS

Renal and Urinary Tract Infections (UTI)

1. Infections can occur within the kidney or the urinary tract. The causative organism also passes into the blood causing a generalized
systemic infection, sepsis or septic shock. Upper tract infections
involve the pelvis of the kidney (pyelonephritis) or the ureters (ure-
teritis). Lower tract infections involve the urinary bladder (cystitis)
or the urethra (urethritis).

   — Risk factors for developing UTI are: (1) an obstruction of the
   urinary tract; (2) reflux flow back into the bladder or up into the
   ureter; (3) invasive procedures into the urinary tract.

2. Escherichia coli is the most common bacterial organism causing
UTI. Other causative organisms are Klebsiella and Proteus. All
of these organisms are normal inhabitants of the colon and fecal
material. They gain entrance to the urinary tract from the perineal
area.

   — Normal emptying of the bladder generally washes out any recent bacterial invaders without any consequence. However,
   when urinary retention occurs, the risk for infectious response
   increases. Retained urine provides a favorable medium for
   bacterial growth and extension of the infectious process upward along the tract and possibly into the blood.

3. Symptoms appear early as the mucosal lining of the bladder is very sensitive. Frequency, urgency, dysuria and hematuria are common signs. Flank pain, fever and chills suggest an upper tract or systemic infection.

    - Examination of the urine for bacteria confirms the diagnosis. A specimen should be sent to the laboratory for culture and sensitivity before antibiotic administration. Most UTIs respond well to antibiotic therapy. Pyridium, an antiseptic, may also be prescribed to relieve the symptoms of burning and urgency.

    - Persons with neurological deficits are at risk for an extension of UTI because they may be unaware of the early signs. Men with benign prostatic hypertrophy (BPH) may also have urinary retention which may lead to extension of UTI. Systemic involvement (fever and chills) may be the first clinical signs identified by person with risk factors. Prompt treatment at the onset of symptoms averts the possibility of sepsis or septic shock.

Bladder Cancer

1. This is the most common carcinoma of the urinary tract. It is usually diagnosed early while it is limited to the bladder because it produces gross hematuria. It occurs most commonly in white men over the age of 60.

2. This oncological condition is treated by surgically removing the growths before the process invades surrounding tissue. Chemotherapy and urinary diversion procedures may be indicated for invasive conditions.

    - Cystectomy is the partial or total removal of the bladder. With partial removal, the bladder capacity is reduced requiring frequent voiding. With total removal, a diversion procedure is performed at the same time.

        • An ileal conduit is a surgical implantation of the ureters into a segment of the ileum which is separated from the intestinal tract. A stoma is created through the abdominal wall which allows continuous urinary drainage into an external collection device.

    - A continent vesicotomy is the surgical creation of urinary control by forming a sealed opening and periodic urinary drainage through the abdominal wall. A catheter is periodically inserted through this artificial sphincter to drain the bladder and thereby providing urinary control. It is an alternative to a neurogenic bladder.

— A nephrostomy is the temporary drainage of urine through a tube placed into the pelvis of the kidney.

Glomerulonephritis

1. This is a disease that affects the glomeruli. Etiological factors are many and varied. They can include (1) immunologic reactions, (2) vascular injury, (3) metabolic disease, and (4) disseminated intravascular coagulopathy.

2. A hemolytic streptococcal infection of the pharynx, tonsil, or skin is the most common underlying site of an infection which may precipatate the disease..

3. In addition to clinical manifestation and laboratory data associated with impaired renal function, the urine appears "smokey" to dark "cola" colored due to marked hematuria and proteinuria. The ASOT titer is elevated indicating the presence of antibodies to streptococcal organism.

4. Usually this is an acute response. If it develops into a chronic state, it may lead to renal failure. A history of glomerulonephritis is the third most common cause of chronic renal failure requiring dialysis.

Stones (Lithiasis)

1. A variety of causes is associated with the formation of stones in the urinary tract; chronic infection, stasis, medications, alkaline urine. Maintaining adequate fluid intake allows the passage of tiny crystals with minimal symptoms. As most urinary stones are irregular in shape, they cause a sudden onset of intense flank pain when they migrate down the ureter or obstruct urinary flow.

2. While most stones are passed, some require surgical removal. Lithotripsy crushes the stone by shock waves or ultrasound.

   — A surgical opening may be made into the obstructed structure to remove the stone. The procedure is named according to the location of the anatomical opening. A pyelolithotomy is the surgical opening into the pelvis of the kidney; whereas the surgical opening into a ureter is called a ureterolithotomy.

   • A tube is placed into the operated structure following surgery to permit urinary drainage. The tube must remain patent as the kidney pelvis can only hold 5 ml. Overdistention leads to damage of the kidney tissue. Accidental removal necessitates return to the operating room for replacement.

Benign Prostatic Hypertrophy (BPH)

1. This is a very common, non-malignant condition which affects 95% of the men over age 70. The cause is unknown but believed to be related to changes in estrogen and androgen levels associated with aging.

2. Because the prostate gland is enclosed within a firm capsule, as it enlarges the diameter of the urethra is compressed. The flow of urine is impaired leading to retention and recurrent UTI. The force of urination progressively decreases, then becomes weak with dribbling. Retention is aggravated by drinking alcoholic beverages, bedrest, other infections, or some medications (decongestants, antidepressants).

   — Symptoms mimic prostatic carcinoma and can be overlooked, ignored or associated with the normal aging process. Serum alkaline phosphatase and prostate-specific antigen (PSA) are tumor marker blood tests that differentiate benign from malignant prostatic enlargement.

3. Surgery is the most common intervention to relieve urinary obstruction.

   — The transurethral prostatectomy (TUR) is the most common approach to restore urine flow. A resectoscope is inserted through the urethra. With continuous flow of sterile saline, segments of the gland are shaved away.

   — Suprapubic prostatectomy involves a lower abdominal incision to remove a larger gland through the bladder. A retropubic prostatectomy involves a similar incision, however the bladder is not entered. These approaches are used when exploration of surrounding tissue is warranted.

4. Following these surgical procedures, there is a risk for hemorrhage or blood clot formation. A large lumen three-way catheter is placed post-operatively to provide continuous irrigation and urinary drainage. Assessment of the color and amount of return fluid is essential. Obstruction in a continuous flow system quickly overdistends the bladder or increases the potential for hemorrhage.

   — The development of blood clots within the bladder irritate the bladder causing spasms. Persons are instructed not to bear down or attempt to pass urine while receiving continuous irrigation. While a sensation to void may be present, straining may increase bleeding from the operative site.

   — After catheter removal, persons are instructed to increase the muscle tone in the perineal area (Kegel exercises). By tightening or squeezing perineal muscles and voluntarily interrupt-

— ing the flow of urine increases bladder control and urine continence.

Renal Failure

1. Renal failure is the inability of the kidneys to adequately filter/
   excrete substances and regulate fluid/electrolyte levels. There
   are two forms: acute or chronic.

   — Acute renal failure (ARF) is generally secondary or a complication of another systemic problem and is potentially reversible.
   Acute tubular necrosis (ATN) is the most common type of
   ARF. It results from acute ischemic or nephrotoxic damage to
   the nephron. Persons with ATN and ARF are usually treated
   in critical care settings where their response to interventions
   can be continuously monitored.

   — Chronic renal failure (CRF) is an irreversible condition which affects all body systems and requires on-going interventions as
   a substitute for physiological renal function. Uremia and end-
   stage renal disease (ESRD) are interchangeable terms. Persons with CRF and other, non-critical medical problems are
   often hospitalized on medical-surgical nursing units. Dialysis
   treatments may be performed at the bedside or on a dialysis
   unit.

   - Malignant hypertension accounts for approximately 25-30%
     of the cases of ESRD. 25-30% of the persons on chronic
     dialysis have Type I diabetes for longer than 10 years. An-
     other 25-30% have a medical history of glomerulonephritis
     or polycystic disease of the kidney. Toxic nephropathy ac-
     counts for 5-10 % of the new cases of ESRD. Based upon
     these figures, the number of new cases of ESRD could be
     decreased with more effective intervention of underlying
     medical problems.

   - Persons with CRF take several categories of medications
     each day: anti-hypertensive agents; diuretics; phosphate
     binding antacids; iron; folic acid; vitamin D; stool softeners;
     calcium supplements, vitamins, cardiotonics. Assessment
     for drug interactions and side effects presents a nursing
     challenge as does the administration of this quantity of tab-
     lets with marked fluid restriction.

   - Persons with CRF are on a special diet which restricts the
     protein intake to daily requirements; limits fluid, sodium and
     potassium intake; high in calories and carbohydrate. The
     diet may also follow diabetic requirements.

- The medical-surgical nurse works closely with the dietitian to determine the appropriate foods/liquids for each person. For example some fruit juices are high in potassium and thus, inappropriate for the diabetic CRF individual who is at risk for insulin shock.

- Liberal use of hard candy is one means to combat the constant thirst and dry mouth experienced by persons with severe fluid restriction. Sugar-free candy is prefered for the diabetic renal patient.

- As erythropoietin activity is diminished with CRF, hematocrit, RBC and hemoglobin values are below normal. It is important to know the individual's parameters. Changes in energy level and fatiguability are subtle indicators of decreasing hematomological values. It is not unusual to observe hematocrit values between 22-25% for a person with CFR and receiving hemodialysis.

2. Hemodialysis is the removal of metabolic waste products and excess water from the body by circulating the blood through a dialyzer (artificial kidney) outside of the body. By regulating the pressure and solutions in the dialyzer, substances move across the dialyzer membrane and are removed.

    — Access to the person's blood is facilitated by the surgical placement of an arterial/venous shunt or central catheter. Patency of these access devices is essential. A shunt is patent when a bruit or thrill is palpated or auscultated over the shunt site. These findings are associated with the turbulence which occurs when venous and arterial blood flow mix.

        - Peripheral blood pressures and blood samples should not be obtained on the extremity with the shunt. Constricting clothing or jewelry on the extremity with the shunt should also be avoided.

        - Assessment of the peripheral circulation and neurological status distal to the shunt is essential. Impaired peripheral blood flow may result as the shunt by-passes or diverts blood from distal anatomy ("steal syndrome").

    — Coordination and cooperation between the nursing staff on the medical-surgical unit and the dialysis staff minimize the occurrence of problems during a dialysis treatment. For example, some medications are removed during dialysis and should be administered after treatment for optimal effect. Other medications potentiate a hypotensive response during dialysis if administered just prior to dialysis.

Focused Bedside Assessment

The following assessment data are associated with the clinical manifestations associated with chronic renal failure with minimal dysfunction of other body systems.

* **General appearance:** Malaise; sallow, yellowish skin color; weak and fatigued; subnormal body temperature; weight loss.

* **Neurological status:** Lethargy; memory impairment; headache; possible seizures; blurred vision.

* **Cardiac status:** Fluid overload; interstitial edema; hypertension; anemia; bounding peripheral pulses; possible ventricular dysrrhythmias (at risk for congestive heart failure); pulsus paradoxus angina.

* **Respiratory status:** Dyspnea; labored breathing; orthopnea; congested lung sounds; possible Kussmaul respirations if severely acidotic.

* **Abdominal (GI) status:** Nausea and vomiting; anorexia; gastritis; stomatitis; metallic taste; thirst.

* **Urinary elimination status:** Progressive decrease in urinary output inspite of fluid intake; unchanging (fixed) urinary specific gravity inspite of fluid intake; foul smelling urine.

* **Extremities:** Dependent edema; paresthesia in the feet; motor weakness; pallor; dry, itchy skin; muscle twitching; petechiae and/or ecchymoses (bruising); peripheral pulses present; noctural leg cramps.

* When the individual is turned on their side, the nurse would expect to find: sacral edema if person is on bedrest; petechiae and/or ecchymoses.

If additional data are observed, a more detailed assessment of the involved system is required. Additional areas of physiological dysfunction may be present and confound the present "renal" problem.

3. Peritoneal dialysis (PD) is the removal of substances from the body by cycling sterile solution in and out of the peritoneal cavity. Substances move from the peritoneal capillaries into the dialyzing fluid and then are drained into collecting devices. Access is achieved through a surgically implanted catheter through the abdominal wall. PD may be accomplished intermittently 2-3 times per week (IPD) or continuously as an ambulatory procedure (CAPD).

   — Individuals on PD are at risk for developing infection (peritonitis). To prevent infections meticulous care is taken during the procedure and with the insertion site. Warning signs of a developing infection include cloudy appearance of the returning solution, temperature elevation above their norm, and chills.

4. Transplantation is a third method of treatment but is not a reality for
    many persons with renal failure. As the availability of donor kid-
    neys is far less than the number of persons with renal failure, only
    persons with no additional body system problems are evaluated
    for potential transplantation. Following transplantation, persons
    will continue immunosuppressive medications in order to prevent
    the development of organ rejection.

    — Signs of rejection include: fluid retention, hypertension, oligu-
       ria, temperature elevation, weight gain, malaise, elevated
       BUN, potassium, creatinine (resembling the onset of renal fail-
       ure). Prompt and aggressive treatment can reverse this re-
       sponse and renal function is restored.

    — Due to the immunosuppressive therapy, these individuals are
       also at risk for superimposed infections from otherwise rela-
       tively non-serious organisms. Fungal (candidiasis) infections
       are particularly troublesome to females.

unit 7

NURSING CARE OF ADULTS WITH

Skeletomuscular Conditions

his unit addresses common recurring conditions of adults which affect body movement and mobility which are often referred to as orthopedic conditions. The care of individuals with skeletomuscular dysfunction on general medical-surgical nursing units is addressed. The management and care of critical and unstable conditions which require continuous monitoring are not addressed in this unit. Examples of clinical situations requiring high acuity care include: fat embolus, unstable multiple fractures, multiple rib fractures with an unstable chest and acute trauma.

SECTION 1: OVERVIEW

Effective plans for care are based upon an understanding of the normal functioning of the skeletomuscular system. This system includes (1) the skeletal framework of the body (bones and joints) which provides support and moveable parts and (2) the soft tissue that provides body movement (muscles, cartilage, fascia, ligaments, tendons and bursae). Movement is necessary to perform normal activity of daily living and is a source of pleasure. There is increasing interest in performing activities that contribute to physical fitness and well-being. When a person's need to move and maintain a desirable body position is altered, other basic human needs and physiological functioning are affected.

Normal Anatomical Considerations

Skeletal framework (bones)

1. 206 bones form the skeletal framework. Each bone is composed of both living cells and nonliving intracellular material. Osteoblasts, osteoclasts and osteocytes are the living bone cells. Bones develop from cartilagineous tissue that undergoes a hardening process with deposits of calcium salts (ossification).

2. There are four types of bones: long (femur, humerus), short (carpals, tarsals), flat (skull, ribs) and irregular (vertebrae, mandible). Each bone is composed of a cancellous (spongy) component and a compact (dense) component. In long bones, the cancellous component is found within the ends or epiphysis. The outer segment of the shaft or diaphysis of a long bone is made of dense, compact component. The center (marrow) of the shaft is porous and contains blood vessels and bone cells.

    — Each bone is surrounded by a fibrous covering (periosteum) to which muscle fibers are attached. The articulating surfaces are covered with cartilage tissue. The epiphyseal line is an adjacent point between the epiphysis and diaphysis.

Joints

1. There are three types of joints: (1) synarthroses which allow no movement (sutures of the skull), (2) amphiarthroses which allow little movement (intervertebral joints) and (3) diarthroses or synovial which allow free movement (hip, knee, shoulder).

2. Each synovial joint contains a small space (joint cavity) between the articulating surfaces of the bone. Articular cartilage which covers the ends of the bone allow for the smooth, gliding motion of the joint. Synovial membrane which lines the capsule provides

the lubricating fluid. The ligaments which are external to the capsule provide joint stability. Small crescent shaped cartilagineous structures (meniscus) provide additional cushioning function.

3. Types of synovial joint movement: hinge (elbow, knee); ball and socket (hip, shoulder); pivot/rotation (wrist, ankle); condyloid, saddle and gliding (hands and feet).

Muscles

1. Muscles are divided into three groups: skeletal (striated, voluntary), visceral (smooth, involuntary) and cardiac. The nerve supply to visceral muscles is supplied by the autonomic nervous system and therefore are involuntarily controlled. Skeletal muscles are innervated by nerves from the cerebrospinal system and control body posture and movement. These striated, skeletal muscles are included in the skeletomuscular system.

2. Striated muscle cells are long and narrow and collectively form muscle fibers. A set of fibers form a muscle mass which is attached between two bones. Muscle masses are located on opposite sides of two bones to produce a balance in movement. For example one set of muscle fibers produce flexion of the forearm toward the shoulder (agonist movement) and another set of fibers produces extension (antagonist movement).

3. Skeletal muscle is very vascular as an adequate blood supply is required for efficient muscle activity. Adequate supplies of oxygen and nutrients especially calcium are required for effective and efficient muscle contraction. The waste products of muscular activity require prompt removal or muscle fatigue and pain occur.

Other skeletomuscular (connective) tissue

1. Cartilage is a firm, gelatinous, avascular tissue that is strong but flexible. Examples include the intervertebral disks and the arti-culating surfaces of bones. Cartilage also provides the anatomical structure to the nose and external ear.

2. Ligaments are bands of dense fibrous connective tissue that areflexible and tough. They connect the articulating ends of bones to provide stability to joints. Ligaments are also located internally to hold anatomical structures in correct position, such as the suspensory ligament which hold the ovary in proximity to the opening of the Fallopian tube.

   — Tendons are bands of dense fibrous extensions of the muscle which attach a muscle to the periosteum of a bone.

3. Fascia is a sheet of loose connective tissue found directly under the skin. Fascia separates one muscle from another to permit independent muscle action.

4. Bursae are small sacs of connective tissue located where pressure is exerted over moving parts. They serve as cushions at the knee, shoulder and elbow joints.

Normal Physiological Functioning

Skeletal framework (bones)

1. Bones provide three mechanical functions: support, protection and movement. In addition, bones provide storage for calcium and the marrow produces red blood cells.

2. Bones heal by a process called callus formation. A hematoma forms from the bleeding fragments of a broken bone or incised segments. Fibroblasts invade the hematoma forming a mesh-work. Then osteoblasts invade to make the meshwork firm. Capillary revascularization develops and delivers nutrients to build collagen. The osteoblasts continue to synthesize new bone within 4-6 weeks.

Muscles

1. The function of muscles is to contract. This is accomplished by a complex process triggered by the transmission of nerve impulses to the muscle fiber. The energy for muscle contraction is supplied by adenosinetriphosphate (ATP) and adenosine diphosphate (ADP) in the presence of calcium ions.

2. The coordination of neural impulse transmission and muscle movement begins in the cerebellum. The fewer number of muscle cells stimulated by a neural impulse, the finer or more precise the muscle movement.

   — At the junction between the neuron and the muscle cell, acetylcholine is released which stimulates the muscle contraction.

3. Types of contractions

   — Isometric contractions increase the tension or tone of the muscles without producing movement.

   — Isotonic contractions are similar and produce movement.

   — Tonic contractions do not produce movement but hold the skeletal framework in position to maintain posture.

   — Twitch is a quick, jerky, involuntary contraction of a small muscle.

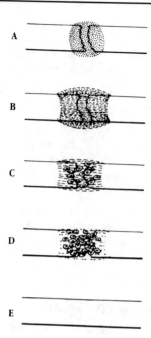

Fig. 7-1. Bone healing (schematic representation). (A) Bleeding at broken ends of the bone with subsequent hematoma formation. (B) Organization of hematoma into fibrous network. (C) Invasion of osteoblasts, lengthening of collagen strands, and deposition of calcium. (D) Callus formation: new bone is built up as osteoclasts destroy dead bone. (E) Remodeling is accomplished as excess callus is reabsorbed and trabecular bone is laid down. From W.J. Phipps, B.C. Long, N.E. Woods: *Medical-Surgical Nursing: Concepts and Clinical Practices*, 5th ed.; St. Louis: Mosby-Year Book, Inc., 1995. Reprinted with permission.

4. Types of movement

   — Flexion refers to moving closer together causing a smaller angle or narrowing space between two bones. For example, bending the knee is flexion. Dorsiflexion refers to moving the toes and foot upward toward the leg causing a small angle between the foot and the anterior aspect of the lower leg. Plantar flexion refers to moving the toes and foot downward and the bottom or plantar surface of the foot is flexed. This movement is opposite to dorsiflexion.

   — Extension refers to moving further apart causing a wider angle or space between two bones. For example, straightening the elbow is extension.

— Abduction refers to movement away from the center of the body. In a similar context, movement of the hands or feet away from center line is called eversion.

— Movement toward the center of the body is called adduction or inversion when this type of movement involves the hands or feet.

— Movement of the hands so that the palms face upward is called supination. This movement relates to the body position (supine) which is recumbent with the anterior surface of the body facing upward.

— Movement of the hands so that the palms face downward is called pronation. This movement relates to the body position (prone) which is recumbent while lying on one's anterior body surface.

Variations Related to Aging

1. Connective tissue progressively loses some of its elasticity and resilience, particularly in the synovial joints and spine. Cartilage becomes more rigid and fragile. Together these changes contribute to the joint stiffness experienced by some elderly.

   — Erosion of the articulating surfaces in synovial joints also leads to joint stiffening especially in the morning of after long periods of inactivity.

2. As vigorous activity decreases, muscles lose bulk, tone and strength which is more evident after age 70. However, age should not be a deterrent to developing an appropriate exercise program for the elderly.

3. Bone reabsorption takes place more rapidly than bone growth. In postmenopausal women, calcium is lost from bone which renders them more porous, thus increasing the risk for fractures.

   — The bone marrow becomes more fatty with a progressive loss of erythropoietin capability. This change contributes to varying degrees of anemia.

4. Loss of cartilage resilience leads to compression of intervertebral disks and increasing the flexion of the spine. This change leads to shortening of body height and flexion curvature of the spine (kyphosis). Increasing flexion of the hips and knees contributes to a more stooped body posture. As the body attempts to compensate for changes in center of gravity, gait and balance are affected. Depending upon the degree of vertebral flexion, respiratory efficiency may be impaired. With these flexion changes, height decreases from 6-10 cm or about 1 inch.

SECTION 2: SKELETOMUSCULAR DYSFUNCTION

Overview

Alterations in the functioning of the skeletomuscular system are related to problems with mobility. Normal anatomy and physiology provide the basis for comparison of symptoms and assessment of findings. Therefore, if the health care provider understands normal findings, the presence of other findings suggest physiological dysfunction and possible pathology.

Assessment of Skeletomuscular Status

1. Performance of activities of daily living (ADL)

   — Information relating to a person's ability to perform daily activities is helpful in determining the extent and nature of nursing interventions required to restore independence. These activities include household, work, recreational and sexual. An individual's perception of the degree of dysfunction is also important. For example, a person may experience noticeable physical impairment and yet conduct most ADL with little assistance. Another person may have little noticeable physical impairment but be unable to participate in essential ADL.

2. Deformity

   Conditions which affect the joints often result in deformity.

   — Kyphosis refers to abnormally increased flexion or roundness of the thoracic vertebral column ("hunch backed").

   — Lordosis refers to abnormal increase in the lumbar vertebral curve ("sway backed").

   — Scoliosis refers to abnormal lateral curvature to the thoracic vertebrae and counter-curvature of the lumbar vertebrae resulting in a S-shaped spinal column. One shoulder is lower and the opposite iliac crest is higher.

   — "Bowed" knees refers to the separation of the knees when the feet are placed together.

   — "Knocked" knees refers to the inability to place one's feet together because one's knees and thighs meet.

   — Contracture refers to the shortening of muscle usually in a flexed position which deceases the range of motion of the involved joint.

3. Strength and range of motion
   – Muscle strength may be graded numerically on a 0 to 5 scale which incorporates muscle contraction and muscle movement. For example, 0/0 means a muscle is paralyzed and there is no visible or palpable contraction. Five/five means full range of active motion against normal resistance.

   – Passive range of motion (PROM) refers to movement of a joint by someone else or a mechanical device

   – Active range of motion (AROM) refers to active movement of a joint by the person with minimal assistance by someone else or a mechanical device.

   – Flaccid refers to less then desired or absent muscle tone.

   – Paralyzed refers to loss of function or voluntary movement. Often altered or loss of sensation accompanies paralysis. "-Plegia" is a word-ending referring to paralysis; whereas "-paresis" is a word-ending referring to marked weakness.

   – "Hemi-" is a prefix to describe involvement on one side of the body

   – "Para-" is a prefix to describe involvement of both lower extremities or below the waist.

   – "Quadri-" is a prefix to describe involvement of all four extremities or below the neck.

4. Sensory changes
   – Dysfunction of the skeletomuscular system often affects peripheral circulation and/or neurological function. Altered or loss of sensation distal to the affected area may suggest secondary neurological impairment.

Diagnostic Testing

1. Various radiographic procedures visualize bone structure such as x-ray and scanning procedures.

2. Joint function is evaluated by scanning and direct visualization:
   – Arthrography refers to the injection of dye into a joint with radiographic visualization. Arthroscopy in the insertion of a small instrument into the joint cavity for direct visualization.

   – The synovial fluid is analyzed (arthrocentesis) for changes in color, clarity, viscosity and cellular elements. Normal synovial fluid is sterile, therefore the presence of any bacteria is indicative of disease.

3. Serum assessment

   — Creatine kinase (CK) concentration is a very helpful assessment of muscle enzymes. CK is normally found in muscle fiber. When disease is present, CK leaks into the serum and levels are elevated.

   — SGOT is a liver enzyme released with various muscle diseases but is non-specific to a skeletomuscular dysfunction.

   — Erythrocyte sedimentation rate (ESR or "sed rate") is increased with inflammatory process which is often associated with joint and muscle conditions. Anti-nuclear antibodies (ANA) titers are also associated with autoimmune joint and muscle conditions.

4. Muscle tissue is excitable and carries an electrical charge. Using sensitive needle electrodes, the electromyogram (EMG) records the potential of muscle fibers to respond or contract.

Measures to Improve Skeletomuscular Functioning

Prevention of dysfunction is the best and most effective intervention to maintain and improve functioning. Good body mechanics are the best preventive action against back injuries. The use of large muscles of the legs for lifting and moving instead of the small back muscles is preventative action.

Interventions to minimize inactivity and immobility will prevent the complications involving other body systems ("disuse syndrome"). For example, with immobility, there is circulatory impairment and the possibility of thrombosis or phlebitis increases. Respiratory activity and elimination become diminished. The risk for skin breakdown increases.

1. Mechanical devices provide support of weakened joints. Splints, braces, assistive devices, such as built up handles on eating utensils, ambulation aids (walkers, canes, crutches) may be helpful.

2. Casts immobilize a broken bone and both joints adjacent to the fractured bone.

   — A short leg walking cast with a cast shoe allows for body mobility with specified skeletal immobility. Synthetic materials to make casts are lighter. Most casts have a stockinette lining to protect the skin surface. If the stockinette becomes wrinkled or other materials lodge between the cast and the skin surface, tissue injury may develop.

— A properly fitted cast does not cause pain or loss of sensation. The portion of the extremity distal to the cast should exhibit normal sensation and movement. Therefore, if pain, underlying pressure or numbness is present, "windowing" or bivalving a cast may be required for restoration of circulatory and/or neurological function.

3. Traction is a mechanism by which a steady, continuous pull is placed on a body part. Countertraction is a force that counteracts the pull of traction. Balanced traction refers to the combination of traction and countertraction to achieve the desired stabilization of a fractured bone.

   — Skin traction is achieved by applying halters, moleskin or adhesive to the skin and attaching a weighted pull to them. Buck's extension, cervical or pelvic halters and Russell traction are examples.

   — Skeletal traction is a weighted pull applied directly to the bone. A pin is surgically inserted through a long bone for weighted attachments. A Thomas splint with a Person attachment is an example of balanced skeletal traction. Crutchfield tongs are inserted into the skull to apply weighted pull for cervical vertebral alignment and immobilization.

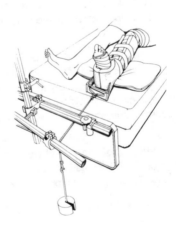

*Fig. 7-2. **Buck's extension.** Heel is supported off bed to prevent pressure on heel, weight hangs free of the bed, and foot is well wawy from footboard of bed. The limb should lie parallel to the bed unless prevented, as in this case, by a slight knee flexion contracture. From W.J. Phipps, B.C. Long, N.F. Woods: Medical-Surgical Nursing: Concepts and Clinical Practices, 5th ed.; St. Louis: Mosby-Year Book, Inc., 1995. Reprinted with permission.*

4. Immobilizing or fixation devices are surgically applied to maintain structures in anatomical alignment or provide physical rest of a damaged part. This hardware includes nails, screws, plates.

5. Replacement parts or prosthesis (refer to Section 3, "Arthritis")
   — Joint replacement

   — Head of the femur replacement

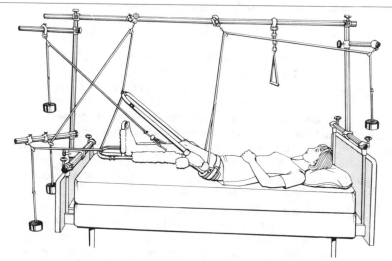

Fig. 7-3. Balanced suspension with Thomas splint and Person attachment. _From W.J. Phipps, B.C. Long, N.F. Woods: Medical-Surgical Nursing: Concepts and Clinical Practices, 5th ed.; St. Louis: Mosby-Year Book, Inc., 1996. Reprinted with permission._

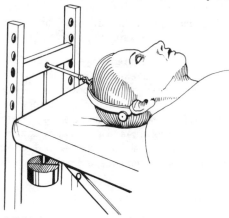

Fig. 7-4. Crutchfield tongs _inserted into the skull are used to maintain traction to the cervical spine. From W.J. Phipps, B.C. Long, N.F. Woods: Medical-Surgical Nursing: Concepts and Clinical Practices, 5th ed.; St. Louis: Mosby-Year Book, Inc., 1996. Reprinted with permission._

SECTION 3: CLINICAL EXAMPLES OF COMMON SKELETOMUSCULAR CONDITIONS

Arthritis

This condition involves an inflammation of one or more joints which may be a chronic systemic condition (rheumatoid arthritis) or secondary to injury (degenerative arthritis or osteoarthritis). Joint pain and stiffness can lead to inactivity and the complications of disuse syndrome. Muscle strength decreases with progressive intolerance to activity.

1. The inflammatory process begins within the joint capsule with edema of the synovial membrane which triggers irritation or damage to the joint tissue (joint swelling). As the process progresses, the articular cartilage and the underlying bone undergoes degenerative changes (pain). Gradually the joint space is narrowed and the articulating surfaces especially in weight bearing joints come in contact with each other (increased pain and joint deformity). Attempts to heal with regenerating articulating surfaces often result in surface irregularity, bone spurs or fusion between surfaces. Chronic pain and dysfunction may result.

   — Osteoarthritis is also known as degenerative joint disease (DJD) which is common especially with increasing age or subsequent to trauma. It is a chronic, progressive condition characterized by increasing localized joint pain, deformity and loss of function. Systemic symptoms of fatigue, fever or other organ involvement are not present. Joint stiffness occurs after periods of rest and improves with activity. Pain is minimized by rest, local heat/hydrotherapy, analgesics, antiinflammatory agents, guided imagery or biofeedback. Larger joints of the knees, hips or spine are commonly affected.

   — Rheumatoid arthritis is a progressive, recurrent, chronic inflammatory arthritis believed related to an altered immune response. With progressive joint involvement, there is considerable subluxation (sliding) joint deformity especially of the hands and feet with subsequent disability. Remissions are achieved with medication: antiinflammatory agents, anti-malarials, injections of medicinal gold salts and corticosteroids. Penicillamine and methotrexate is used if other approaches are ineffective.

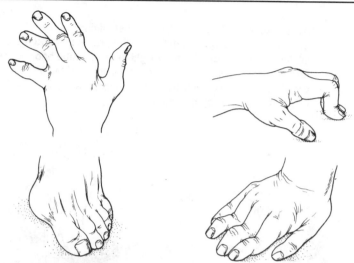

Fig. 7-5. Typical deformities of rheumatic arthritis. _From W.J. Phipps, B.C. Long, N.F. Woods: Medical-Surgical Nursing: Concepts and Clinical Practices, 5th ed.; St. Louis: Mosby-Year Book, Inc., 1996. Reprinted with permission._

- Gouty arthritis is a specific type of crystal-induced arthritis which results from elevated serum uric acid levels and abnormal deposits of uric crystals in the joints of the feet, toes and vertebrae. An acute inflammatory attack may be precipitated by serious illness, acute stress, cancer chemotherapy, alcohol ingestion or end-stage renal disease. Specific medications are used to lower serum uric acid levels: colchicine, probenecid, sulfinpyrazone or allopurinol.

3. Joint replacement may be indicated when the pain and dysfunction is severe and not responding to non-surgical management. To minimize the possibility of infection, antibiotics are administered before surgery and for several days post-operatively. Infection of the replacement may require the removal in which case there is non-union at the operative site or no functional joint.

   - Knee replacement or total knee arthroplasty (TKA) involves the surgical removal of the articulating surfaces of the femur and tibia. Synthetic replacement parts are cemented to the bone ends. Tendons and ligaments are secured around the joint for stabilization. Specific activity and restrictions are coordinated with physical therapy personnel.

   - Hip replacement or total hip arthroplasty (THA) involves the replacement of the acetabulum and the head of the femur with an interfemoral shaft. To prevent dislocation, patient needs to be instructed in the following: to keep the leg abducted (out to the side) at all times; to avoid internal rotation and keep leg in a neutral position; to avoid acute flexing of hip (caution patient not to exceed a 90 degree angle when sitting). Adduction or internal rotation causes tension on the prosthesis and the possibility of dislocation. Partial weight-bearing ambulation is preferred to sitting which places undue flexion and tension on the prosthesis. Specific activity and restrictions are coordinated with physical therapy personnel.

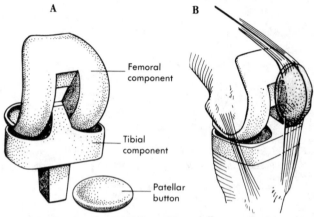

A   B

Femoral
component

Tibial
component

Patellar
button

Fig. 7-6. Knee replacement: (A) Tibial and femoral components of total knee prosthesis. (B) Total knee prosthesis in place. From W.J. Phipps, B.C. Long, N.F. Woods: Medical-Surgical Nursing: Concepts and Clinical Practices, 5th ed.; St. Louis: Mosby-Year Book, Inc., 1995. Reprinted with permission.

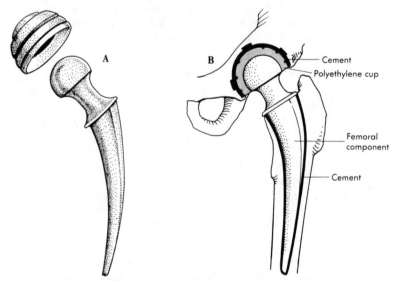

A   B   Cement
                                         Polyethylene cup

                                         Femoral
                                         component

                                         Cement

Fig. 7-7. Hip replacement: (A) Acetabular and femoral components of total hip prosthesis. (B) Total hip prosthesis in place. From W.J. Phipps, B.C. Long, N.F. Woods: Medical-Surgical Nursing: Concepts and Clinical Practices, 5th ed.; St. Louis: Mosby-Year Book, Inc., 1995. Reprinted with permission.

Osteomyelitis

This condition is an acute or chronic infection of a bone. The source of microorganism invasion may be from a compound fracture, a penetrating wound or orthopedic surgery. It may also develop from extension from soft tissue infection, such as ischemic, diabetic or neurotropic ulcers.

1. Clinical manifestations include pain in the involved area, fever, malaise and possible signs of sepsis. X-rays may reveal areas of radiolucency (osteonecrosis) 2-3 weeks after the onset of the process. These areas of devitalized bone become separated from the surrounding healthy bone forming islands of infection. Blood-borne antibiotics and leukocytes have difficulty penetrating an established area of osteomyelitis to facilitate healing. Surgical debridement may be required before antibiotic therapy can be effective.

2. Antibiotic therapy is required for 6 weeks to 3 months. Open, draining areas may be irrigated or packed with antibiotic products. On-going monitoring for toxic effects of long-term antibiotic therapy is required.

   − Aminoglycosides: gentamicin, kanamycin, neomycin, streptomycin, tobramycin have the risk for ototoxicity (decreased hearing, dizziness, ringing sound), nephrotoxicity (raising BUN and creatinine levels), or superimposed infections from loss of normal bacterial flora.

   − Penicillins: ampicillin, methacillin, oxacillin have the risk for anemia, hypersensitivity (hives, dermatitis) and overgrowth of nonsusceptible organisms.

   − Cephalosporins: cefazolin, cephalothin, cefoxitin have the risk for photosensitivity, increasing BUN, hepatotoxicity (elevated enzymes; SGOT, SGPT, LDH, jaundice), colitis and overgrowth of nonsusceptible organisms.

Fractures

A fracture is a break in the continuity of a bone. It occurs when physiologic stress or pull is placed on the bone which exceeds the bone's capacity to endure. Trauma is the most common cause. Pathologic fractures occur when the physiologic stress or pull is within normal limits but the bone capacity is decreased. This abnormal state occurs with diseased bone, such as osteoporosis or neoplasms. Osteoporosis and fractures are quality of life issues for the elderly.

1. A suspected fracture is treated as though a fracture is present until it is ruled out. Interventions include immobilization of the affected bone and adjacent joints, elevation of the affected area, local application of ice, and assessment of circulatory and neurological status distal to the injury.

2. Fractures are treated by three methods:

    — Closed reduction is the manipulation of displaced fragments into their normal anatomical alignment which is maintained by immobilization until healing occurs. Traction, casts and splints are methods of immobilizing the area.

    — Open reduction and internal fixation (ORIF) is indicated for unstable fractures or when prolonged bedrest and traction would not be well tolerated. Internal fixation is accomplished by the surgical insertion of nails, screws, wires, pins, plates or bone grafts.

    — External fixation consists of the surgical insertion of skeletal pins that penetrate the fracture fragments and attach to an external frame to provide stabilization and immobilization.

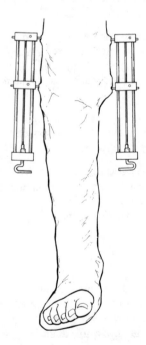

Fig. 7-8. External fixator. From W.J. Phipps, B.C. Long, N.F. Woods: Medical-Surgical Nursing: Concepts and Clinical Practices, 5th ed.; St. Louis: Mosby-Year Book, Inc., 1995. Reprinted with permission.

3. With fractures that protrude through the skin surface or following ORIF, there is risk for infection of the soft tissue (cellulitis) or of the bone (osteomyelitis).

   – Meticulous care of the incision and hardware insertion sites will minimize the possibility of infection and protocols may vary with physicians and institutions. Insertion site care usually includes daily cleansing of the site, possible removal of any accumulated crusts and the application of antibacterial ointment.

   – Signs of persistent redness, swelling, drainage or increased pain may indicate an infection. Culture and sensitivity of the drainage should be obtained before the initial administration of antibiotics.

4. Fractures of long bones have a risk for the development of fat embolism in which fragments of the bone marrow are released into the general circulation. This complication is most likely to occur within 72 hours of the fracture incident but may occur up to 10 days post injury.

   – An embolus travels through the venous system and lodges in the pulmonary vasculature. Sudden onset of anxiety, tachycardia, tachypnea, profuse tracheobronchial secretions and petechial rash involving the conjunctiva, trunk and neck warrant immediate intervention.

   – Depending upon the degree of cardiopulmonary involvement, the patient may be transferred to a critical care setting for continuous cardiac and hemodynamic monitoring and continuous anticoagulant therapy.

5. Compartment syndrome is an acute complication involving edema and soft tissue injury secondary to a fractured long bone. Compression of tissue within fascia walls may impair blood flow with increasing risk of muscle ischemia and neurological deficit.

   – Clinical manifestations include progressive pain distal to the injury with inability to extend digits. The overlying skin appears normal because surface vessels are not compressed. Other symptoms may include numbness, tingling and diminished peripheral pulses.

   – The extremity should be elevated with the application of cold/ice to the involved area. Constricting bandages, casts or traction may require readjustment. Surgical incision of the fascia may be required for severe compression (fasciotomy).

6. Fractured hip is a somewhat inaccurate wording as the hip is a joint and therefore cannot be fractured. The skeletal parts that may be fractured are the greater trochanter, the neck of the femur or the head of the femur.

— The blood supply to this part of the body and the location of the fracture dictates the treatment. The major source of blood supply enters below the neck of the femur and extends laterally down the trochanter and upward into the neck and head of the femur. Therefore, if a fracture occurs below the source of blood supply (intertrochanteric fracture) the fractured parts can be nailed together (internal fixation). However, if the fracture occurs in the neck of the femur, the blood supply will be disrupted and avascular or aseptic necrosis of the head of the femur will develop. In this situation, the prosthetic head of the femur with an intramedullary shaft will be inserted into the femur. This procedure is commonly refered to as "hip surgery" and should not be confused with a total hip replacement.

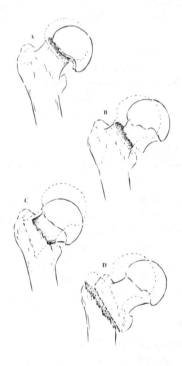

Fig. 7-9. Fractures of the hip: (A) subcapital fracture; (B) transcervical fracture; (C) impacted fracture of base of neck; (D) intertrochanteric fracture. From W.J. Phipps, B.C. Long, N.F. Woods: *Medical-Surgical Nursing: Concepts and Clinical Practices,* 5th ed.; St. Louis: Mosby-Year Book, Inc., 1995. Reprinted with permission.

Focused Bedside Assessment

The following assessment data are associated with the clinical manifestations associated with an acute fracture of the hip with minimal dysfunction of other body systems.

* **General appearance:** Acute intense pain usually at the lateral aspect of the involved hip; pain is more intense if the leg is moved; signs of shock often present.

* **Neurological status:** Attention is focused on the source of the pain.

* **Cardiac status:** Secondary tachycardia which minimizes with pain relief.

* **Respiratory status:** Secondary, shallow tachyapnea which minimizes with pain relief.

* **Abdominal status:** WNL.

* **Urinary elimination status:** WNL.

* **Extremities:** Outward rotation of the foot on involved side; peripheral pedal pulses and capillary refill to toes should be similar to unaffected side unless peripheral circulation is impaired; affected side leg is shorter.

* When the individual is turned on their side, the nurse would expect to assess no unusual findings, but the person does not tolerate being turned as the pain intensifies.

If additional data are observed, a more detailed assessment of the involved system is required. Additional areas of physiological dysfunction may be present and confound the present "orthopedic" problem.

Amputation

This procedure is required for certain conditions, such as severe peripheral vascular disease, severe orthopedic trauma, and malignant bone tumors. Today, most amputations are performed for advanced peripheral circulatory impairment and gangrene in the lower extremities, especially in diabetic persons over 60 years of age. Unless the underlying cause that is necessitating the amputation is controlled, there is increased mortality rate. It is estimated that there is less than a 50% five-year survival of persons following a lower extremity amputation.

1. When progressive peripheral vascular impairment is present, some physicians recommend peripheral bypass surgery to improve the circulation proximal to the involved area. Femoral-popliteal procedure usually increases the peripheral circulation to the lower leg and foot. This procedure is often recommended prior to an amputation to improve the circulatory status to the stump. Improved circulation may make a difference between and above the knee (AK) and below the knee (BK) amputation.

2. The choice of removal procedure depends upon the area of the limb involved. The surgical goal is to remove the least amount of tissue possible while achieving optimal circulation to remaining tissue and thereby healing of the stump. Sometimes it may appear that considerable tissue is removed with a BK amputation when only an infected toe is observable. Vascular studies usually indicate severe arterial impairment to the foot that would not permit adequate healing if only the infected area was removed.

3. Postoperatively, the stump is elevated. A closed drainage system such as a Hemovac or Duval may be placed under the skin flaps to minimize the accumulation of fluid at the operative site.

    — The stump may be wrapped or placed in a cast or temporary prosthesis to prevent edema and to facilitate molding. Monitoring the stump tissue is required to ensure circulatory adequacy. The capillary refill should be less than two seconds. Skin surface should feel warm and exhibit the person's normal skin color (similar to the non-amputated extremity).

    — Early ambulation and arm strengthening exercises are advocated to prevent flexion contractures and loss of muscle strength. This effort also promotes positive psychological outlook and improves circulatory functioning and wound healing.

    — Phantom limb sensations may occur following surgery and may persist for several months. Phantom pain is often perceived as intense to the person following surgery as the preoperative pain. Chronic preoperative conditions tend to produce persistent phantom pain. The nerves that transmit the pain sensation continue to transmit similar impulses even though the source of the pain was removed. During the immediate postoperative period it is difficult to differentiate between actual and phantom pain. As healing occurs, relief of phantom pain is usually achieved by local massage, heat, biofeedback techniques or TENS (transcutaneous electrical nerve stimulation). Occasionally, surgical exploration of the stump to resect a neuroma or to resect the involved nerve is required for pain relief.

    — If the stump is inadequately treated, it may become edematous and is more prone to injury which will delay the fitting of a prosthesis. If loss of sensation is present, the risk of skin breakdown on the stump remains.

Disuse Syndrome

An immobilized person is at risk for alterations in the functioning of many body systems. The potential dysfunction is presented according to the problems to be prevented.

1. Impaired skin integrity
   - The risk for skin breakdown results from prolonged compression of soft tissue between a bony prominence and an underlying contact surface. Shearing movement, moisture and malnutrition increase the risk. Numerous mattresses, overlays and specialty beds are available to redistribute pressure over a wider body surface. Meticulous skin care and frequent change of position are essential interventions to prevent skin breakdown.

2. Altered respiratory function
   - Diminished ventilatory capacity and retained secretions lead to atelectasis and hypostatic pneumonia. Routine use of incentive inspirometer promotes adequate deep breathing and aeration of most segments of the lung.

3. Muscle atrophy
   - Loss of muscle mass and tone develops from disuse and inactivity. Active range of motion of joints not immobilized and isometric muscle-setting exercises minimize the loss of muscle mass and strength.

4. Impaired peripheral circulation
   - With muscle atrophy and inactivity, there is diminished intermittent external compression of the veins to facilitate venous return. Without this activity, venous stasis occurs and the risk for thrombus formation increases.

5. Bone demineralization
   - With decreased muscle activity, there is decreased physical tension or weight-bearing stress on the bones (disuse osteoporosis). Calcium moves from the bones into circulation (hypercalcemia).

6. Constipation problems are usually corrected by increased fluid and dietary fiber intake.

7. Urinary stasis
   - With prolonged supine, recumbent position, normal physiological gravity-flow drainage of the urinary tract does not occur. Stasis of urine in the bladder or kidney pelvis develops. If an indwelling catheter is required, the risk for ascending urinary tract infection increases. If bone demineralization occurs, elevated serum calcium levels result. The potential for stone formation increases as the urinary calcium levels rise.

unit 8

NURSING CARE OF ADULTS WITH

Special Needs

T *his unit addresses the special care needs of adults who have conditions which affect the dysfunction of more than one body system. The care of these individuals occurs on general medical-surgical units. The management and care of critical and unstable situations involving these conditions which require continuous monitoring are not addressed. The special needs addressed in this unit include: care during the perioperative cycle, care of adults with oncological conditions, and care of adults with altered immune responses.*

SECTION 1: NURSING CARE OF ADULTS DURING THE PERIOPERATIVE CYCLE

The perioperative cycle includes the preoperative, intraoperative and immediate postoperative periods. While specific aspects of care of individuals experiencing various surgical procedures were included in the appropriate body system units, this section addresses essential aspects common in the care of all surgical procedures.

Perioperative Care

1. Advance directives are written guidelines stating a person's directions for their care if they are in a position in which they are no longer able to make those decisions. A person, usually the next of kin, is named as the individual who is authorized to make decisions on their behalf.

    — If the person has a living will, it should be placed in the record.

2. Informed consent (operative permit) is the signed and witnessed permission to perform the stated surgical procedure. Prior to signature, a full explanation of the procedure and specific tissues to be removed is provided in terms easily understood by the person. The possible complications and risk of death associated with this procedure are explained and stated in the permission form. This explanation is provided by the primary physician and/or the surgeon.

    — Nursing personnel assess and verify the individual's understanding of the surgical procedure and the potential complications. The nursing staff reinforce and clarify the individual's understanding. Appropriate translation into the individual's primary language and level of understanding is essential. Diagrams, models or other audiovisual aids may be used for clarification. Explanations should be clear and concise without overloading the individual with excess information.

    — If a misunderstanding exists, the physician or surgeon is contacted for further clarification. Surgery may be postponed.

3. An explanation of the sequence of events that will occur reassures the individual and alleviates unnecessary anxiety related to the fear of the unknown. Some institutions have videos of pre-operative events for the person and their families. Information on visiting hours and location of waiting rooms are appreciated by families. If it is anticipated that the individual will be spending some time in a special care unit after surgery, visiting that unit and meeting the personnel are helpful.

4. Persons who will experience long surgical procedures or who are at risk for peripheral vascular impairment are fitted for anti-embolic or pneumatic compression stockings. Isometric leg exercises are demonstrated and practiced.

Focused Bedside Assessment

The following assessment should be completed prior to administering the prescribed preoperative medication. Many institutions have specific documentation forms which are completed before transfer to the OR.

* **General appearance:** Anxious behavior varies with individuals from calm, relaxed and joking manner to mild restlessness and tenseness. Extreme anxiety or fear requires re-evaluation by the surgeon. High anxiety is associated with rapid and disconnected speech, asking questions without waiting for answers and not finishing sentences. These persons may be diaphoretic with cold and clammy hands, tachycardic, tachypneic and often hyperventilate while talking.

* **Neurological status:** WNL. Verify and document the quality of sleep the night before surgery. All artificial prostheses are removed, such as false eyes, hearing aids, removable dental work, contact lenses. Sensory disabilities such as blindness or hard of hearing, are clearly documented on the record for other healthcare providers obtaining assessment data.

* **Cardiac status:** A preoperative EKG is obtained on persons with a history of cardiac disease or over age 40. Results are included in the chart. Usually a complete blood count is required.

* **Respiratory status:** Chest x-ray is taken on all persons who will receive general anesthesia with results placed in the chart. As cigarette smoking irritates lung tissue, data on smoking activity during the 24 hours prior to surgery is obtained. The presence of "cold-like" symptoms are reported to the anesthesiologist and recorded in the chart.

* **Gastrointestinal status:** NPO unless otherwise ordered. Bowel sounds are present but diminished. A history of alcohol or substance abuse is reported and recorded.

* **Urinary elimination status:** The time and amount of the voiding immediately prior to the preoperative medication is recorded. Routine urinalysis should be in record.

* **Extremities:** WNL. Nail polish is removed for optimal visualization of peripheral circulation. All jewelry is removed and given to the family. The identification band is securely placed on the individual.

* **Other data:** The results of laboratory work should be on the chart when they are transported to the operating suite. Abnormal findings should be reported to the surgeon.

— Other postoperative activities, procedures and equipment are demonstrated and practiced preoperatively. Deep breathing and coughing activities, use of the incentive in spirometer, movement in and out of bed are examples of preoperative activities.

Recovery Room (RR) or Post-Anesthesia Care Unit (PACU)

1. Upon the arrival of a person from the operating suite to a recovery care unit, an initial assessment occurs. The sequence begins with the basic ABC (airway, breathing and circulatory status) and then proceeds with the assessment of other body system function. The following assessment data provides a guideline for this initial activity following general anesthesia.

2. Focused Initial Postoperative Bedside Assessment

* Positioning for an adequate airway and breathing. For the person who is spontaneously breathing and is semi-conscious, an oral airway is used to hold the tongue in place. The possibility of airway obstruction is minimized. The head is placed to one side with the chin extended if there is a problem with tongue placement. Supplemental oxygen is administered by cannula or mask.

* Vital signs are taken every five minutes x 4. If stable and within the range that occurred during surgery, assessment of vital signs extends to every 15 minutes and then every 30 minutes. The cause of any deviation is promptly identified.

* All intravenous lines, drains, urinary catheter and other equipment noted on the operative record are located and assessed for function. The incisional area is examined for unusual findings and to establish the baseline for future comparison of data.

* Neurological status: The person progressively arouses and responds appropriately to orientation questioning, then quickly returns to a sleeping state with no sense of time lapsed. Restless movement is an early indicator of incisional and operative pain. Raised siderails are required safety precautions.

* Cardiac status: Tachycardia may be present especially with acute pain and following specific types of anesthesia. Elevated systolic blood pressure is common with acute pain and agitated behavior. Analgesia is beneficial but may cause hypotension. Dysrhythmias may indicate tissue hypoxia, hypoventilation, response to specific anesthetic agents or hypovolemia. Hypotension may be related to a rapid change in body position during the transfer process, fluid or blood loss or response to analgesia especially following meperidine (Demerol) administration.

* Respiratory status: Breath sounds are clear or comparable to the preoperative status. Assessment of peripheral tissue oxygenation by an oximeter is common. SaO_2 values above 90% are desirable to ensure adequate tissue oxygenation and cellular metabolism (80% is the minimum).

* Gastrointestinal status: Diminished functioning with no or minimal audible bowel sounds.

* Urinary elimination: Urinary output should equal fluid intake. Optimal hourly urinary output should be above 50 ml. Minimal acceptable urinary output for an adult is 30 ml/hour. Refer to Unit 6 for additional discussion on acute renal insufficiency.

* Extremities: The skin usually feels cold and some persons experience the cold with shivering. External warmed linen is often provided to facilitate the return of body temperature to normal parameters. Peripheral pulses are equal and present.

3. Management of care following regional or spinal anesthesia

    — Regional anesthesia is produced by injecting an anesthetic agent along the course of a nerve thus abolishing impulse transmission to and from the area supplied by that nerve. The anesthetic agent is usually introduced into the subarachnoid space between lumbar 3-4 vertebral level.

    — The person experiences no pain in the anesthetized area and remains awake. Usually sedation is administered to alleviate the anxiety and stress associated with being overaware of one's surroundings. The operative area is screened from the person's vision but conversation and activities among operating room personnel are heard and remembered.

    — Regional or spinal anesthesia is not used for operating on the upper part of the body because it causes paralysis of the diaphragm and intercostal muscles. Respiratory effectiveness is impaired with levels of anesthesia involving the thorax.

    — Vasodilation often occurs below the level of anesthesia and may result in varying degrees of hypotension. Anti-embolic stockings minimize the severity of this problem.

    — Sensation usually returns within 1-2 hours following surgery. Refer to the dermatome chart in Unit 1 for further understanding of spinal nerve innervation of peripheral sensation and muscle activity.

    — A headache may occur following spinal anesthesia and is minimized by hydration, remaining flat for several hours and using a dimly-lighted environment. Analgesics are helpful. This side effect diminishes with no long-term effects.

— The assessment of return of sensation and movement are obtained and the time recorded. When there is complete return of sensation in the toes (in response to pinprick) and voluntary movement, the person is usually considered to have recovered from the effects of spinal anesthesia.

4. The person is ready to transfer from this immediate postoperative care unit when there is evidence of recovery from the anesthesia, vital signs are stable and there is no untoward effects from surgery or the anesthesia.

— This evaluation is crucial when the person will be transferred out of the hospital. Most institutions will not permit the operated person to leave unaccompanied. Detailed care instructions are provided to both the person and their home- care provider or family member. Instructions also include the procedure for contacting the physician or institution if questions or problems develop. All instructions are documented on the record at time of discharge or transfer.

Care During the Postoperative Period

1. Stabilization of the circulatory system

— Hemorrhage is a possibility within 48 hours following surgery. Due to the trauma of surgery, small vessels at the operative site are vasoconstricted and in vasospasm. As the effects of anesthesia diminish, these vessels relax which may result in bleeding. Consequently, post-operative hemorrhage may be delayed for several hours. Bleeding is not always apparent from the incision when internal bleeding occurs. Increased incisional pain, agitation, falling blood pressure, increasing pulse rate and decreasing urinary output are indicators of internal bleeding.

— Various anesthetics and analgesics are known to produce varying degrees of peripheral vasodilation. When compared to pre-operative parameters, a low blood pressure and elevated pulse rate often indicate inadequate fluid replacement. Stabilized blood pressure and pulse values accompanied by an adequate urinary output are indicators of stabilized circulatory status.

— Sudden changes in body position or acute pain often alters hemodynamic stability. Intermittent peripheral vasodilation may occur producing changes in the blood pressure, pulse rate or urinary output.

— Ice chips are administered as the first source of oral fluids when the person is fully awake. Assessment for bowel

sounds, abdominal distention and nausea determine a
person's tolerance of oral intake. For tabulation of intake and
output, approximately two cups of ice chips is equivalent to
one cup of liquid. If fluid intake is not adequate, a low-grade
fever will develop.

— Adequate replacement of fluid loss is required during the NPO
state. If the person is NPO longer than 24 hours, then potassium replacement is considered and added to the daily IV fluids. Potassium is found in adequate amounts in most foods
but is not stored in the body. Therefore, daily requirements of
potassium are provided.

Guidelines for IV potassium administration:

* Determine the adequacy of urinary output before IV potassium replacement is initiated.

* The flow rate of IV fluids with potassium should not exceed 10-20
mEq/hour or in concentrations greater than 30-40 mEq/Liter of
fluid.

* Potassium is irritating to vessels and causes some discomfort during administration. A slow infusion rate in peripheral vessels is
better tolerated.

* Potassium is also very irritating to subcutaneous tissue. Therefore, infiltration may result in tissue necrosis.

2. Respiratory adequacy

— Incisional pain may decrease a person's ability and desire to
breath deeply or cough sufficiently to expel secretions from the
respiratory track. Areas of hypoventilation may lead to collapse of alveoli or atelectasis. The regular use of an incentive
inspirometer facilitates adequate aeration of the lungs. Also,
encourage coughing and deep breathing at least every four
hours while awake.

— Due to the irritating effects of general anesthesia, excess pulmonary mucus production often occurs. Retained secretions
and hypoventilation may produce a low-grade fever during the
early postoperative period.

3. Adequate healing and prevention of infection

— An adequate nutritional state prior to surgery is the best predictor of effective wound healing. Vitamin C and protein are
needed for tissue repair. If delayed oral intake is anticipated,
hyperalimentation is initiated as a preventative intervention of
nutritional deficiencies.

- Incisions are closed with sutures, wires, staples or tape. Only a small dressing or incisional covering is used. If there is not drainage, the operative dressing will be removed within 24-48 hours.

- Any disruption in the skin surface provides an entrance for microorganism invasion. Therefore, a draining incision is a source for potential infection to the person or to others if the wound drainage is contaminated. Tubes and drains placed near the incision remove any accumulation of drainage beneath the skin surface but also provide a route for microorganism invasion.

- Good handwashing before and after the care of a wound is essential for preventing infections. Sterile technique is used for all care of the dressing or incision. Dressings and equipment used for incisional care are treated as if contaminated.

- Antibiotic therapy may be administered before, during and after surgery when an infected procedure is anticipated. Preventive antibiotic therapy is also administered in situations where the risk for postoperative infection is high (intestinal procedures) or the complication of an infection would undermine the procedure (joint replacement). In these situations, the clinical signs of infections are masked.

- If an incision does not adequately heal, the edges separate (wound dehiscence). If the degree of incisional separation is extensive the underlying tissue protrudes (wound evisceration). Warm, moist, sterile compresses are applied to the area until the surgeon examines it.

4. Convalescence and discharge instructions
   - With the occurrence of early discharge, ambulatory surgery and increasing elderly population, the need for providing effective discharge instructions becomes imperative. Identifying the need for home health care services is an increasing responsibility of the bedside nurse. Planning for continuity of care and adequate referral minimize the incidence of hospital readmission within two weeks of discharge.

   - Self-care instructions prior to discharge include verbal and written materials with a clearly stated name and phone number for individuals to contact the physician or hospital if questions arise. Persons often do not realize the problems that they may encounter until they are in the situation. Many hospitals provide telephone follow-up within the first 24 hours after "day" or ambulatory surgery.

— During normal healing, the edges of a non-infected, dry surgical incision are sealed within 48 hours. For this reason, incisional dressings are usually removed during this time frame. During the next 4-5 days, fibroblasts infiltrate the incisional area and internal healing begins. Capillary proliferation and lymphatic drainage are re-established. Cellular regeneration occurs. It takes an additional 4-5 weeks for the collagen structure to become established with firm scar tissue formation. This process may be lengthened for some healing, such as intracranial healing, draining or infected wounds, bone infections or when selected microorganisms are involved.

— Certain activities may be limited during the 4-6 week convalescent period in order to promote adequate rest and decrease strain on the operative site, especially following an abdominal incision. For example, heavy lifting is often limited to objects weighing less than a gallon of milk. Climbing stairs may also be limited in the number of steps or the number of times per day. Restrictions on driving a car limits a person's physical activity and encourages physical rest.

— Fatigue is an expected reaction; however, exhaustion should be avoided especially with the current trends of early hospital discharge. Often for 4-6 weeks following major surgery, the person may not experience "getting tired" and only experience feeling well or exhausted. The perception of becoming tired is diminished for some persons during this convalescent time frame. Planned rest periods throughout the day and adequate nighttime sleep minimize the occurrence of exhaustion. Persons should be informed that endurance of activities progressively increases.

Management of Pain

1. Pain is a symptom which also exhibits some objective indicators.

   — Nonverbal indicators of pain include: grimace or tension of facial muscles; restlessness and irritability; increased skeletal muscle tension; sleep disturbance.

   — Systemic or autonomic indicators of pain include: diaphoresis; vasoconstriction (pallor); increased blood pressure; increased pulse rate; pupillary dilation; mild hyperglycemia.

2. Analgesic medications may be administered by injection, intravenously, orally or by intermittent self-administration. Side effects include respiratory depression, sedation, nausea and vomiting. Meperidine may also cause excitement and hypoten-

sion. Naloxone (Narcan) should be available to reverse the occurrence of severe respiratory depression.

— Intramuscular injection analgesia is the most common route of administration for moderate to severe pain. Morphine, meperidine (Demerol), pentazocine (Talwin), nalbuphine (Nubain), butorphanol (Stadol), burenorphine (Buprenex) are often prescribed to be administered 3-4 hours prn. There is a possibility of excessive sedation. Toradol may be prescribed for 48 hours to reduce the need for narcotics.

— Analgesia by intravenous bolus is prescribed for severe, intermittent pain. This route of administration produces rapid onset of pain relief for a short duration. Morphine or meperidine (Demerol) is helpful prior to painful procedures or treatments.

— Oral preparations are useful for mild to moderate pain relief. This route cannot be used until the GI tract is functioning. Codeine, oxycodone (Percodan), meperidine (Demerol), propoxyphene (Darvon) are commonly prescribed preparations. Non-narcotic and nonsteroidal inflammatory preparations are also effective for mild to moderate pain; such as acetominophen (Tylenol), ibuprofen (Motrin, Advil, Nuprin), indomethacin (Indocin), naproxen (Naprosyn, Anaprox), and ketorolac (Toradol).

— Patient-controlled analgesia (PCA) is useful for moderate to severe pain. This approach enables titration in which predetermined dosages administered by the patient without the possibility of overmedication. It has been found that lower dosages are required to achieve desired analgesia. Meperidine (Demerol) or morphine are used, but Dilaudid is frequently used by terminally ill patients..

3. Non-pharmacologic methods may be effective independently or in association with medication to control pain.

— Back and foot massage relax muscular tension and increase local circulation. However, calf pain should not be massaged as a circulatory problem may be present.

— Transcutaneous nerve stimulation (TENS) send weak impulses via electrodes placed on the body. The sensation of chronic pain is often reduced.

— Limiting anxiety increases a person's pain tolerance. Explanation of anticipated events, progressive relaxation techniques and slow controlled deep breathing are helpful in many situations. Guided imagery is another technique in which mental images are employed to promote relaxation and decrease pain sensations.

4. Abdominal procedures which involve manipulation of intestinal structures tend to cause a delay in the return of peristalsis (ileus). Pockets of air within the intestine tend to cause intermittent cramping "gas" pain. Physical activity (walking) tends to facilitate the passage of "gas." The passage of flatulence is associated with intact gastrointestinal functioning.

5. Air trapped within the peritoneal cavity tends to rise and rests against the diaphragm during the immediate postoperative period. The irritation causes sharp pain which often radiates to unoperative locations; such as the shoulder. The air is gradually absorbed within 1-2 days without any residual problems.

SECTION 2: NURSING CARE OF ADULTS WITH ONCOLOGICAL CONDITIONS

Overview

Perhaps over the past 30 years, no other disease has caused more fear and disability than cancer. Today, it remains the second leading cause of death among adults in the United States. Tremendous strides have been made in the methods of early detection which have increased the five-year survival/cure rate for many types of malignancies. It is estimated that today the number of persons alive and symptom-free or without recurrence five years after the initiation of treatment ("cure rate") is almost 50%. For some types of cancers, such as early-stage Hodgkin's disease and testicular cancer, the statistics approach 60-90%. However, for lung cancer the survival rate is only 13%. Therefore, with current trends, cancer should be considered a chronic illness rather than an inevitable lethal event.

1. Tumors or neoplasms are abnormal growths which may be benign, malignant or metastatic.

   — Benign tumors usually resemble the tissue of origin, are encapsulated and do not invade surrounding tissue. They may become problematic because increasing tumor size causes pressure or compression of neighboring organs.

   — Malignant tumors include cells which have undergone structural changes resulting in pathophysiological differences from the tissue of origin. They are not well defined and invade surrounding tissue.

— Metastatic tumors are abnormal growths which result from the migration of tumor cells to a new location via the circulatory or lymphatic systems. These secondary growths resemble the primary lesion in their pathophysiology rather than the tissue at the new location. Metastatic growths are not well defined and invade surrounding tissue.

2. Tumors are described by anatomic site and tissue origin. Carcinomas and adenomas arise from epithelial tissue. Carcinoma in situ refers to localized or pre-invasive epithelial tumors. Sarcomas arise from connective tissue. Lymphomas arise from lymphatic tissue. Gliomas arise from glial cells of the central nervous system. Leukemias arise from blood-forming organs. Melanomas arise from pigment cells.

3. Tumor grading is an evaluation of a tumor's degree of malignancy or degree of spread beyond the primary site.

4. Tumor staging determines the extent of the disease in an individual.

Management of Care

The overall aim of cancer management is to cure the malignancy. When this is not possible, the aim is to control its growth in order to extend the person's useful life. These aims are accomplished by surgery, radiation, chemotherapy and on-going supportive care. The coordination of treatment regimes are usually discussed at tumor boards, which are organized committees with representation of the primary physicians, medical specialists and oncology nurses.

1. Surgical removal is the treatment of choice when the tumor is localized with no known metastasis. The procedure includes the removal of the tumor with sufficient surrounding tissue to include any tissue invasion and regional lymph nodes which may contain micrometastases. The tumor is carefully removed to minimize the inadvertent loss of tumor cells into the circulatory system.

   — Palliative or non-curative procedures may be performed to control metastatic spread or to relieve difficult and obstructive symptoms. For example, the removal of a bleeding, necrotic tumor may provide physical comfort for a person. And, a bowel resection may remove an obstructive tumor, restore physiological function and allow the person to resume eating.

2. The aim of radiation therapy is the eradication of malignant cells without producing excessive toxicity or damage to normal tissue. It can be used alone or in combination with surgery or chemotherapy. When used in combination with another mode of treatment, the approach is referred to as adjuvant radiation. Radiation may

also be used palliatively to control bone metastases, reduce pain and decrease the risk of fractures.

— Radiation therapy is delivered by three approaches: (1) an external beam to an internal target (the tumor); (2) the implantation of a radioactive substance into the tumor; or (3) the systemic administration of a radioactive isotope which migrates and accumulates at the cancer site. With the development of sophisticated equipment, external radiation is used more commonly that other modes. There now is less tissue-damaging effects than reported in the past.

3. Chemotherapy is the administration of antineoplastic drugs in a systemic or regional manner to cure or control a malignancy. It is an adjuvant therapy used in combination with surgery or radiation. While significant toxicities are associated with this treatment, it has the advantage of reaching undetected micro- metastases.

— Chemotherapeutic agents or cytotoxic drugs are classified according to their action of specific phases of cell growth and reproduction. Alkylating agents, such as carmustine, cisplatin, dacarbazine, Cytoxan, nitrogen mustard. Antibiotics include bleomycin, doxorubicin (Adriamycin), mitomycin C. Antimetabolites include 5 Fluorouracil, methotrexate. Plant alkaloids include vinblastine, vincristine (Oncovin).

— A combination of agents is often used and administered in a dosage and treatment schedule to maximize the contact with vulnerable cells. Successful treatment regimes and schedules usually produce side effects on different body system and do not have additive effects. The more toxic drugs are administered in a cyclic pattern over a longer time frame. Other drugs have greater tumoricidal effect with initial doses than with repeated doses.

— Because most of these drugs are toxic substances, health care providers are advised to complete an approved course. Most agents require specific procedures for safe preparation, handling, administration and disposal of administration equipment.

Supportive Nursing Care

1. Venous Access Devices (VAD) are frequently used to minimize the trauma of multiple venipunctures and the possibility of tissue damage from infiltrated chemotherapy. Catheters or ports (Hickman, PortaCath, Broviac) are surgically implanted in a central vein under local anesthesia. Specific instructions on dressing care,

flushing techniques and cap-changing routines are essential prior
to home care.

- Because most agents are very irritating and damaging to soft
  tissue, care is essential to prevent contact. Special care is required if intravenous access is used to prevent extravasation.
  Patency of peripheral access is established with isotonic solutions prior to chemotherapy administration.

2. Management of side effects is an on-going effort. Most chemotherapeutic agents affect cells that reproduce quickly. Certain normal
   cells are also affected resulting in varying degrees of side effects.

   - Bone marrow suppression leads to neutropenia, thrombocyto-
     penia and anemia. The risk for opportunistic infections in-
     creases as well as spontaneous bleeding. Prompt reporting of
     a fever, chills, nosebleed or tarry stool facilitates appropriate
     early intervention.

   - As the epithelial tissue is also affected, varying degrees of nau-
     sea, vomiting and diarrhea often occur. A combination of vari-
     ous antiemetics, tranquilizers and antihistamines are
     administered at scheduled intervals 12 hours before, during
     and following chemotherapy. Cold or room temperature foods
     are tolerated better than hot, aromatic foods. Clear liquids
     and bland foods taken in small amounts and at frequent inter-
     vals are usually tolerated.

   - Stomatits is a side effect associated with bleomycin, metho-
     trexate and 5-Fluorouracil. The symptoms of taste alterations
     and ulceration also impair oral intake. Good oral hygiene with
     a water-pik and non-alcohol mouthwash reduce oral debris.
     Local anesthetics provide comfort. Nystatin preparations con-
     trol secondary fungal infections.

   - Alopecia (hair loss) is another distressing side effect. The psy-
     chological impact affects individuals differently. Care to pro-
     tect the head from cold exposure and direct sun is essential.

3. Facilitating effective coping skills and acceptance are essential.
   Fighting cancer is an emotional battle as well as a physical one.
   Learning to cope with the change in one's future and loss of control over one's life requires a variety of strategies. In addition to
   one's personal past experiences and coping skills, support systems are essential. Primary nursing care provides for continuity of
   care during and after hospitalization which is built upon established rapport.

   - Provide information as requested in concise and readily under-
     stood words. Avoid bombarding the person and their family
     with a wealth of information. Correct misconceptions as they
     arise.

- Repeating information is common as the person is often pre-occupied with their feelings and have decreased concentrations. Repeated questions may be a way one seeks validation of their understanding.

- Encourage the person to share their thoughts and feelings. Be prepared for expressions of anger, tearful sadness, isolation and confusion. Hope and seemingly unrealistic expectations are often a form of protection of one's self and significant others. The person will come to terms with reality in their own way according to their time frame and ability to cope with the changes occuring in their lives. Health care providers are available for realistic encouragement as the person faces everyday challenges.

- Encourage participation in support groups and individual counseling for specific concerns. Religious support and counseling may be helpful.

SECTION 3: NURSING OF ADULTS WITH ALTERED IMMUNE CONDITIONS

Overview

Our body protects itself from injury and invasion of foreign materials or microorganisms. Intact skin and mucous membranes of the respiratory, gastrointestinal and urinary tracts are the first barriers. The normal bacteria (flora) on the skin and secretions of the glands of the skin discourage the growth of disease producing microorganisms (pathogens). The body attempts to get rid of invaders by mechanical clearance. For example, foreign or harmful materials can be coughed out of the respiratory tract, vomited from the gastrointestinal tract or flushed through the urinary tract.

If there is a break or cut in the skin or mucous membrane, invading pathogens trigger internal responses which complement each other. The first response is the inflammatory response which begins within seconds of an injury or invasion. The affected tissue is soon surrounded with white blood cells and fluid. The invader is isolated, destroyed or removed. Then healing occurs.

The next line of defense, immunity, occurs more slowly and is a systemic response specific to an invader or antigen. Long-term protection can be gained by specific cellular responses and the production of antibodies. Natural immunity occurs when the body recognizes an invader and produces an appropriate antigen-antibody response. Acquired immunity occurs from therapeutics interventions, such as vaccinations or exposure to and recovery from certain diseases.

Hypersensitivity

1. Sometimes the sophisticated response to a foreign substance breaks down causing the immune system to react inappropriately. The exaggerated response to an environmental substance or antigen is one example.

   - Persons at risk for severe reactions should wear Med-Alert identification.

2. Hypersensitive reactions are classified as "immediate" when systemic manifestations appear within minutes of exposure. A delayed response may take several hours before symptoms appear and re-exposure may produce a more severe reaction. Anaphylaxis is a rapid, severe and sustained response which does not respond to the usual interventions and is considered to be a medical emergency.

3. The clinical manifestations are attributed to the biologic effects of histamine on the tissues of the gastrointestinal tract, skin and the respiratory tract.

   - Gastrointestinal hypersensitivity is frequently manifested by vomiting, diarrhea and abdominal pain. Foods most frequently implicated include milk, chocolate, citrus fruits, eggs, wheat, nuts, peanut butter and seafood. Sometimes the allergen is not the food but the drug, additive or preservative in the food.

   - Skin manifestations of allergic responses are primarily urticaria (hives) and occur in response to local contact or injection of an allergen. White, fluid-filled blisters surrounded by areas of erythema or redness are the typical response. Varying degrees of itching (pruritis) are experienced.

   - Effects of allergens on the mucosa of the eyes, nose and respiratory tract are well-known and experienced by the general population. The manifestations of conjunctivitis, rhinitis and other "cold-like" symptoms are troublesome. However, when the inflammatory response and mucosal edema lead to bronchospasm, the situation becomes more severe. If the signs of expiratory wheezing progress to include inspiratory stridor, gas exchange becomes impaired. An acute asthmatic attack may warrant the continuous administration of bronchodilating medication which may precipitate cardiac dysrhythmias. Continuous care and monitoring in a critical care setting may be required until the symptoms are controlled.

4. Refer to Unit 3 for additional information and the discussion of the care of asthma.

Autoimmune Response

1. Intolerance to one's own tissue and self antigens is described as an autoimmune response and is another inappropriate response made by our immune system. Isoimmunity is a similar response in which an individual reacts against other human tissue as in the cases of rejection of transplanted tissues and sperm allergies.

2. Several conditions have been linked to an autoimmune response as the causative factor: systemic lupus erythematous (SLE), Graves' disease (a thyroid dysfunction), hemolytic and pernicious anemias, myasthenia gravis and rheumatoid arthritis.

Acquired Immune Deficiency Syndrome (AIDS)

Acquired Immune Deficiency Syndrome (AIDS) is a life-threatening illness caused by the human immunodeficiency virus (HIV). A person who is positive for HIV but does not have symptoms of AIDS has "HIV Disease." This may or may not develop into AIDS in the future. The person is, however, a lifelong carrier of HIV and is able to transmit the virus to others. In addition, a person can be infected with the virus and be negative in blood testing, especially in the early stages of infection. Although HIV has been found in the blood as early as one week after exposure, the majority of cases seroconvert between 6 and 18 weeks (95% within 3 months, 99% within 6 months).

HIV has been isolated from blood, semen, vaginal secretions, saliva, tears, breast milk, cerebrospinal fluid, amniotic fluid, and urine, but epidemiological evidence has implicated only blood, semen, vaginal secretions, spinal fluid, and breast milk in transmission. However, the CDC recommends that barrier precautions be used for all body fluids except sweat. The low levels of HIV in these fluids does not mean that HIV cannot be transmitted through them, but the number of viruses present in the fluid is so small that the risk of infection is minimal. The human behaviors believed to be directly involved with the transmission of HIV are as follows:

— Intercourse with an infected person

— Sharing needles with an infected person

— An infected woman to her baby during pregnancy

— Getting blood transfusions of infected blood (a lower risk since blood screening began in 1985)

Stages of Illness Progression

AIDS is a disease of the immune system. The virus invades and destroys the white blood cells that fight infection. The official diagnosis of AIDS is not made until the helper T-cell count falls below 200. However, the T-cell number does not always tell how sick a person is. Some persons with fewer than 200 T-cells seem quite healthy while others with higher counts are already suffering from opportunistic infections.

The viral load (measurement of HIV in circulation) is an accurate predictor of severity of illness and survival. Persons with lower viral loads have a greater chance of survival. Currently, viral load of less than 5000 indicates a favorable long-term outcome. There are four stages of HIV infection:

1. Acute infection

   This stage occurs in up to 70% of all infected individuals. During this time, blood tests will begin to show antibodies to the virus (3-8 weeks after infection). Reported symptoms indicating this stage are flu-like with sweating, generalized red rash, and difficulty breathing. The symptoms typically last 2-4 weeks and disappear without treatment.

2. Clinical Latency

   This stage begins as the body successfully cleanses itself of the virus and traps it in the lymph nodes. While in the lymph nodes, the virus makes copies of itself. In response, the body makes antibodies which neutralize any HIV particles left in circulation and produces specialized white blood cells (killer T-cells) which attack and destroy infected tissue. An infected person can remain in this stage from 6 months to over 10 years. The virus continues to replicate but at a much slower rate than it does in acute infection (Stage 1). The person is healthy and carries out all daily activities normally.

3. Chronic phase

   This stage can last anywhere from months to years. Viral replication increases and CD4 cells decrease. The individual becomes symptomatic with fever, weight loss, malaise, pain, fatigue, loss of appetite, abdominal discomfort, diarrhea, night sweats, headaches, and swollen lymph glands. The ability to carry out normal daily activities may be impaired. The degree of impairment varies from one day to the next.

4. AIDS

Of the persons in Stage 3, above, about 30% will develop AIDS related infections within 5 years. In this stage there is rapid viral replication and depletion of the immune system. In addition to the symptoms in Stage 3, the person may develop malignancies, opportunistic infections and develop toxicity to the drugs used to combat HIV and AIDS.

— Drug therapy is esential in the treatment of HIV and AIDS patients. However, the drugs attack only the virus that is produced in the body each day and cannot eliminate the virus that was present before drug therapy was started. Also, the drugs must be taken exactly as ordered or resistance develops quickly. Current treatment with combination therapy (3 or more drugs) is geared toward using different drugs, each of which attacks a different part of the HIV virus that is produced. By attacking the virus on multiple fronts, it also takes longer for drug resistance to develop. Multiple drug therapy also helps to minimize dose-related side effect.

— In order to be diagnosed with AIDS, and HIV patient must also meet one or more of the following criteria:

- The CD4+T lymphocyte count drops below 200/mm^3.

- The development of one of the following opportunistic infections (OIs):

  ° Fungal: candidiasis of bronchi, trachea, lungs or esophagus; disseminated or extrapulmonary histoplasmosis

  ° Viral: Cytomegalovirus (CMV) disease other than liver, spleen or nodes; CMV retinitis (with progressive loss of vision); herpes simplex with chronic ulcer(s) or bronchitis, pneumonitis or esophagitis; progressive multifocal leukoencephalopathy (PML), extrapulmonary cryptococcosis.

  ° Protozoal: disseminated or extrapulmonary coccidioidomycocis, toxoplasmosis of the brain, Pneumocystis carinii pneumonia (PCP), chronic intestinal isosporiasis; chronic intestinal cryposporidiosis.

  ° Bacterial: Mycabacterium tuberculosis (any site); any disseminated or extrapulmonary Mycobacterium, including *M. Avium* complex or *M. Kansasii*; recurrent pneumonia; recurrent *Salmonella* septicemia.

- The development of one of the following opportunistic cancers: invasive cervical carcinoma, Kaposi's sarcoma (KS),

---

Focused Bedside Assessment

The following assessment data are associated with the clinical manifestations related to AIDS with minimal dysfunction of other concurrent, pre-existing or unrelated pathophysiological conditions.

* **General appearance:** Recurrent fever, cachexia; herpes infections; dermatitis; fungal infections of the skin, mouth and perineum; enlarged lymph nodes.

* **Neurological status:** Flattened affect; apathy; memory deficits; recurrent headaches.

* **Cardiac status:** Tachycardia; friction rub; gallops; murmurs.

* **Respiratory status:** Tachypnea; dyspnea; diminished or adventitious sounds (crackles, rhonchi, wheezes); dry cough.

* **Gastrointestinal status:** Chronic and recurrent diarrhea; enlarged liver or spleen.

* **Urinary elimination:** May be incontinent.

* **Extremities:** Unsteady gait; dermatitis of skin of extremities; joint and muscle pain; muscle atrophy.

         Burkitt's Lymphoma, immunoblastic lymphoma, or primary lymphoma of the brain.

  • Wasting syndrome occurs. Wasting syndrome is defined as a loss of 10% or more of ideal body mass.

  • Dementia develops. AIDS-related dementia causes neurocognitive deficits and behavioral symptoms that are not related to other causes.

Modified from: Centers for Disease Control and Prevention (CDC). (1992, December 18). Recommendations and Reports: 1993 revised classification system for HIV infection and expanded surveillance case definition for AIDS among adolescents and adults. Morbidity and Mortality Weekly Report, 41 (RR-17), 1-17

Infection control interventions

The goal of infection control is to prevent the transmission of HIV from the person to health care providers and from one person to another person via a health care provider. In addition, interventions focus on activities to prevent the transmission of potential harmful organisms to the immune deficient person.

  — Disposal of needles and "sharps" at the bedside in puncture proof containers minimize the possibility of injury and exposure of the virus to health care providers. Do not attempt to recap a needle before disposal.

In 1996, the Centers for Disease Control and Prevention revised their recommendations for preventive practices. These new precautions, called Standard Precautions, require the use of barrier equipment for any contact with blood, body fluid (except sweat), mucous membranes, nonintact skin, secretions, and excretions. Gloves should be worn during suctioning and oral hygiene. They are not needed when feeding unless you have reason to believe that your hands will contact secretions or mucous membranes. Gloves, gowns, masks, and eyewear are used to protect the health care provider if contact with blood, body fluid, secretions, excretions, mucous membranes, or nonintact skin is likely. This protects the health care worker from personally acquiring the virus, and avoids inadvertently carrying it to another person at another bedside. Effective and appropriate handwashing is essential.

High efficiency particulate air respirator filter (HEPA) masks, or the equivalent N95 or PFR95 respiratory filter are worn in cases of active tuberculosis. The ventilation system in the isolation room is modified to a negative pressure environment. Drug resistant strains of a mycobacterium tuberculosis have been identified among HIV and AIDS infected persons.

— Protective eyewear is advocated for care and treatment activities that have the potential for splashing of body fluids on health care providers.

— Immune suppressed persons should avoid activities with large groups where the possibility of exposure to infectious microorganisms is high. Contact with individuals with the common cold should also be avoided.

— Self-care measures to maintain skin integrity are essential, such as daily hygienic care using mild, nondrying soap. Avoid prolonged pressure on bony prominences. Daily oral hygiene maintains intact mucous membrane.

1. Interventions to manage the chronic and incapacitating effects of muscle (myalgia) and joint (arthralgia) pain accompanied by progressive weakness and fatigue.

— Biofeedback technique, diversional activities and relaxation exercises increases one's pain tolerance. Slow, soothing music with slow, deep breathing often provides relaxation and increases pain threshold.

— Administer analgesic and muscle relaxant medication as prescribed.

— Refer to Section I of this unit for additional information on pain management and use of analgesics.

2. Foster optimal acceptance of a life-threatening condition by encouraging the person to express their feelings.

   — Provide positive feedback with a focus on facts rather than the myths and misconceptions.

   — Encourage access to counseling and support groups.

   — Support patient and significant others through anticipatory grieving.

   — For more information, contact the AIDS Hotline:
   1-800-342-AIDS (2437)
   1-800-334-7432 (Spanish)
   1-800-243-7889 (TTY)

Appendix

The 1996-97 List of NANDA Nursing Diagnoses

- Activity Intolerance
- Activity Intolerance, Risk for
- Adaptive Capacity, Decreased Intracranial
- Adjustment, Impaired
- Airway Clearance, Ineffective
- Anxiety
- Aspiration, Risk for
- Body Image Disturbance
- Body Temperature, Risk for Altered
- Breastfeeding, Effective
- Breastfeeding, Ineffective
- Breastfeeding, Interrupted
- Breathing Pattern, Ineffective
- Cardiac Output, Decreased
- Caregiver Role Strain
- Caregiver Role Strain, Risk for
- Communication, Impaired Verbal
- Community Coping, Ineffective
- Community Coping, Potential for Enhanced
- Confusion Acute
- Confusion, Chronic
- Constipation
- Constipation, Colonic
- Constipation, Perceived
- Coping, Defensive
- Coping, Ineffective Individual
- Decisional Conflict (Specify)
- Denial, Ineffective
- Diarrhea
- Disuse Syndrome, Risk for
- Diversional Activity Deficit
- Dysfunctional Ventilatory Weaning Response
- Dysreflexia
- Energy Field, Disturbance

- Environmental Interpretation Syndrome, Impaired
- Family Coping, Compromised, Ineffective
- Family Coping, Disabling, Ineffective
- Family Coping, Potential for Growth
- Family Processes, Altered
- Family Processes, Altered; Alcoholism
- Fatigue
- Fear
- Fluid Volume Deficit
- Fluid Volume Deficit, Risk for
- Fluid Volume Excess
- Gas Exchange, Impaired
- Grieving, Anticipatory
- Grieving, Dysfunctional
- Growth and Development, Altered
- Health Maintenance, Altered
- Health-Seeking Behaviors (Specify)
- Home Maintenance Management, Impaired
- Hopelessness
- Hyperthermia
- Hypothermia
- Incontinence, Bowel
- Incontinence, Functional
- Incontinence, Reflex
- Incontinence, Stress
- Incontinence, Total
- Incontinence, Urge
- Infant Behavior, Disorganized
- Infant Behavior, Potential for Enhanced Organized
- Infant Behavior, Risk for Disorganized
- Infant Feeding Pattern, Ineffective
- Infection, Risk for

- Injury, Risk for
- Knowledge Deficit (Specify)
- Loneliness, Risk for
- Management of Therapeutic Regimen, Effective, Individual
- Management of Therapeutic Regimen, Ineffective, Community
- Management of Therapeutic Regimen, Ineffective, Family
- Management of Therapeutic Regime, Ineffective, Individual
- Memory, Impaired
- Noncompliance (Specify)
- Nutrition: Less than Body Requirements, Altered
- Nutrition: More than Body Requirements, Altered
- Nutrition: Potential for More than Body Requirements, Altered
- Oral Mucous Membrane, Altered
- Pain
- Pain, Chronic
- Parent/Infant/Child Attachment; Risk for Altered
- Parental Role Conflict
- Parenting, Altered
- Parenting, Risk for Altered
- Perioperative Positioning; Risk for Injury
- Peripheral Neurovascular Dysfunction, Risk for
- Personal Identity Disturbance
- Physical Mobility, Impaired
- Poisoning, Risk for
- Post-Trauma Response
- Powerlessness
- Protection, Altered
- Rape-Trauma Syndrome
- Rape-Trauma Syndrome: Compound Reaction
- Rape Trauma Syndrome: Silent Reacon

- Relocation Stress Syndrome
- Role Performance, Altered
- Self-Care Deficit: Bathing/Hygiene, Dressing/Grooming, Feeding, Toileting
- Self-Esteem, Chronic Low
- Self-Esteem, Situational Low
- Self-Esteem Disturbance
- Self Mutilation, Risk for
- Sensory/Perceptual Alterations (Specify: Visual, Auditory, Kinesthetic, Gustatory, Tactile, Olfactory)
- Sexual Dysfunction
- Sexual Patterns, Altered
- Skin Integrity, Impaired
- Skin Integrity, Risk for
- Sleep Pattern Disturbance
- Social Interaction, Impaired
- Social Isolation
- Spiritual Distress (Distress of the Human Spirit)Suffocation, HighRisk for
- Spiritual Well-Being; Potential for Enhanced
- Swallowing, Impaired
- Thermoregulation, Ineffective
- Thought Processes, Altered
- Tissue Integrity, Impaired
- Tissue Perfusion, Altered (Specify Type: Renal, Cerebral, Cardiopulmonary, Gastrointestinal, Peripheral)
- Tissue Perfusion; Altered Cardiac
- Trauma, Risk for
- Unilateral Neglect
- Urinary Elimination, Altered
- Urinary Retention
- Ventilation, Inability to Sustain Spontaneous
- Violence, Risk for: Self-Directed or Directed at Others

INDEX

Other Publications From
Skidmore-Roth Publishing, Inc.

	CODE	ISBN #	PRICE	QTY
INSTANT INSTRUCTOR SERIES				
AIDS/HIV	ADIN01	1-56930-010-0	$ 16.95	
C.C.U.	CCINC1	1-56930-022-4	$ 16.95	
Diabetes	DBII01	1-56930-041-0	$ 16.95	
Geriatric	GRN01	0-944132-68-5	$ 16.95	
Hemodialysis	DLIN01	1-56930-020-8	$ 16.95	
I.C.U.	ICUI01	1-56930-021-6	$ 16.95	
IV	IVII01	1-56930-043-7	$ 16.95	
Lab	LBIN01	0-944132-70-7	$ 16.95	
Obstetric	OBIN01	0-944132-67-7	$ 16.95	
Oncology	ONIN01	1-56930-023-2	$ 16.95	
Pediatric	PDIN01	0-944132-66-9	$ 16.95	
Psychiatric	PSY101	0-944132-69-3	$ 16.95	
NURSING CARE PLANS SERIES				
AIDS/HIV	ADSC01	0-56930-000-3	$ 36.95	
Critical Care	CNCP01	1-56930-035-6	$ 36.95	
Geriatric (2nd ed.)	GNCP02	1-56930-052-6	$ 36.95	
Oncology	ONCP01	1-56930-004-6	$ 36.95	
Pediatric (2nd ed.)	PNOP02	1-56930-057-7	$ 38.95	
SURVIVAL SERIES				
Geriatric Survival Handbook	GSGD01	1-56930-061-5	$ 29.95	
Nurse's Survival Guide (2nd ed.)	NSGD02	0-944132-75-8	$ 29.95	
Obstetric Survival	OBSG01	0-944132-94-4	$ 29.95	
Pediatric Survival Guide	PNGD01	1-56930-018-6	$ 29.95	
RN NCLEX REVIEW SERIES				
Concepts of Medical Surgical Nursing	NMS01	0-944132-85-5	$ 21.95	
Concepts of Obstetric Nursing	NOB01	0-944132-86-3	$ 21.95	
Concepts of Psychiatric Nursing	NPSY01	0-944132-83-9	$ 21.95	
PN/VN Review Cards (2nd ed.)	PNRC02	1-56930-008-9	$ 29.95	
RN Review Cards (2nd ed.)	RNRC02	0-944132-82-0	$ 29.95	

Other Publications From
Skidmore-Roth Publishing, Inc.

	CODE	ISBN #	PRICE	QTY
NURSING/OTHER				
Body in Brief (3rd ed.)	BBRF03	1-56930-055-0	$ 35.95	
Diagnostic and Lab Cards (2nd ed.)	DLC02	0-944132-77-4	$ 27.95	
Drug Comparison Handbook (2nd ed.)	DRUG02	1-56930-16-x	$ 35.95	
Essential Laboratory Mathematics	ELM01	1-56930-056-9	$ 29.95	
Geriatric Long-Term Procedures & Treatments	GLTP01	0-944132-97-9	$ 34.95	
Geriatric Nutrition and Diet (2nd ed.)	NUT02	1-56930-045-3	$ 19.95	
Long Term Care, A Skills Hand-book (2nd ed.)	HLTC02	1-56930-058-5	$ 23.95	
Handbook for Nurse Assistants (2nd ed.)	HNA02	1-56930-059-3	$ 23.95	
I.C.U. Quick Reference	ICQU01	1-56930-003-8	$ 32.95	
Infection Control	INFC01	1-56930-051-8	$ 99.95	
Nursing Diagnosis Cards (2nd ed.)	NDC02	1-56930-060-7	$ 29.95	
Nurse's Trivia Calendar, 1998	NTC98	1-56930-073-9	$ 11.95	
OBRA (2nd ed.)	OBRA02	1-56930-046-1	$ 99.95	
OSHA Book (2nd ed.)	OSHA02	1-56930-069-0	$ 119.95	
Procedure Cards (3rd ed.)	PCCU03	1-56930-054-2	$ 24.95	
Pharmacy Tech	PHAR01	1-56930-005-4	$ 25.95	
Spanish for Medical Personnel	SPAN01	1-56930-001-1	$ 21.95	
Staff Develop for the Psych Nurse	STDEV0	0-944132-78-2	$ 59.95	
OUTLINE SERIES				
Diabetes Outline	DB)L01	1-56930-031-3	$ 23.95	
Fundamentals of Nursing Outline	FUND01	1-56930-029-1	$ 23.95	
Geriatric Outline	GER01	0-944132-90-1	$ 23.95	
Hemodynamic Monitoring Outline	HDMO01	1-56930-034-8	$ 23.95	
High Acuity Outline	HATO01	1-56930-028-3	$ 23.95	
Medical-Surgical Nursing Outline (2nd ed.)	MSN02	1-56930-068-2	$ 23.95	
Obstetric Nursing Outline (2nd ed.)	OBS02	1-56930-070-4	$ 23.95	
Pediatric Nursing Outline	PN01	0-944132-89-8	$ 23.95	

Name _____

Address _____

City _____

State _____ Zip _____

Phone (   ) _____

    ❑ VISA   ❑ MasterCard   ❑ American Express

    ❑ Check/Money Order

Card # _____ Expiration Date _____

Signature (required) _____

Prices subject to change. Please add $6.95 each for postage and handling. Include your local sales tax.

Mail or Fax your order to:

SKIDMORE-ROTH PUBLISHING, INC.
2620 S. Parker Road, Suite 147
Aurora, Colorado 80014
1 (800) 825-3150 -- FAX (303) 306-1460

or

Visit our website at: http://www.skidmore-roth.com